Rotator Cuff Injury Explained.

Including Rotator Cuff Tear, Rotator Cuff Bursitis, Rotator Cuff Tendonitis.

Symptoms, Exercises, Stretches, Repair, Recovery, Aids, Treatments, Alternative Therapies all covered.

by

Robert Rymore

Published by IMB Publishing 2013

Foreword

My friend Graham was diagnosed with Rotator Cuff Tear and he wanted to know more about it. That is the reason why I wrote this book.

I love giving people information about medical conditions in order to help them.

Table of Contents

Chapter 1) Introduction

This book is an explanatory guide to your rotator cuff injuries. The causes, risk factors and the mechanism of injuries are discussed in detail in this book. More than that, it focuses on the treatment side of the rotator cuff injuries. Non-surgical management, surgical management as well as postoperative management for each rotator cuff injury type is mentioned descriptively in the subsequent chapters.

Before diving in deep, it is worth knowing some vocabulary used in this book regarding the movements of the shoulder joint.

1) Movements of the Shoulder

Shoulder abduction:	Raising the arms sideways
Shoulder adduction:	Lowering the arms sideways
Shoulder flexion:	Raising the arms forward
Shoulder extension:	Moving the arm backward
Shoulder medial rotation:	Taking the arm behind back
Shoulder lateral rotation:	Turning the arm out sideways

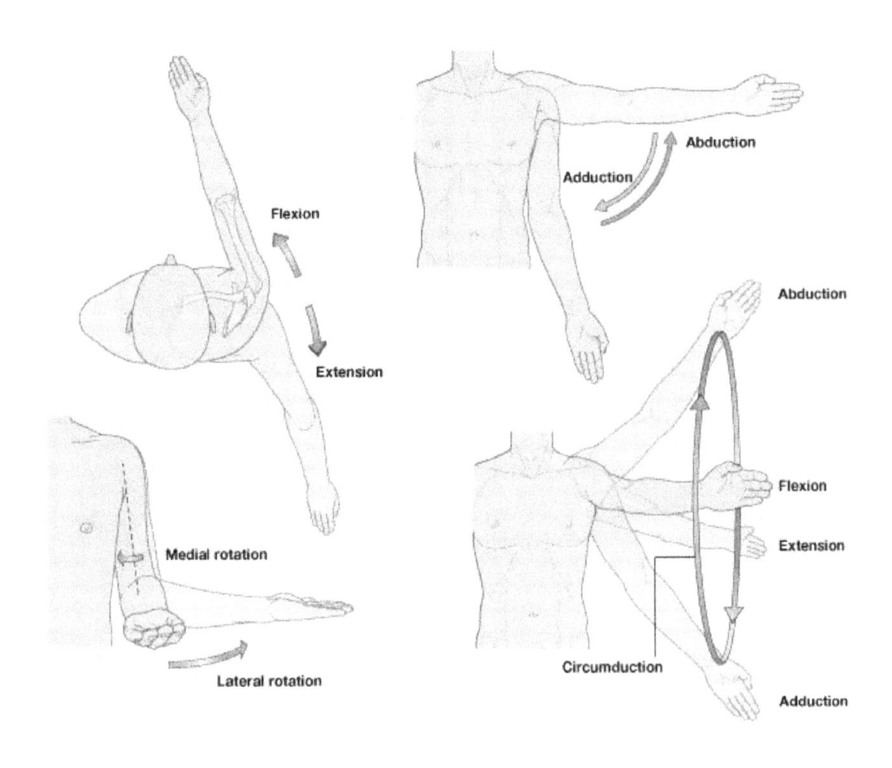

2) Movements of the Scapula (Shoulder Blade)

Shoulder elevation: Shrugging of the shoulder

Shoulder depression: Dropping of the shoulder

Shoulder protraction: Moving the shoulder forward

Shoulder retraction: Squeezing of the shoulder blade

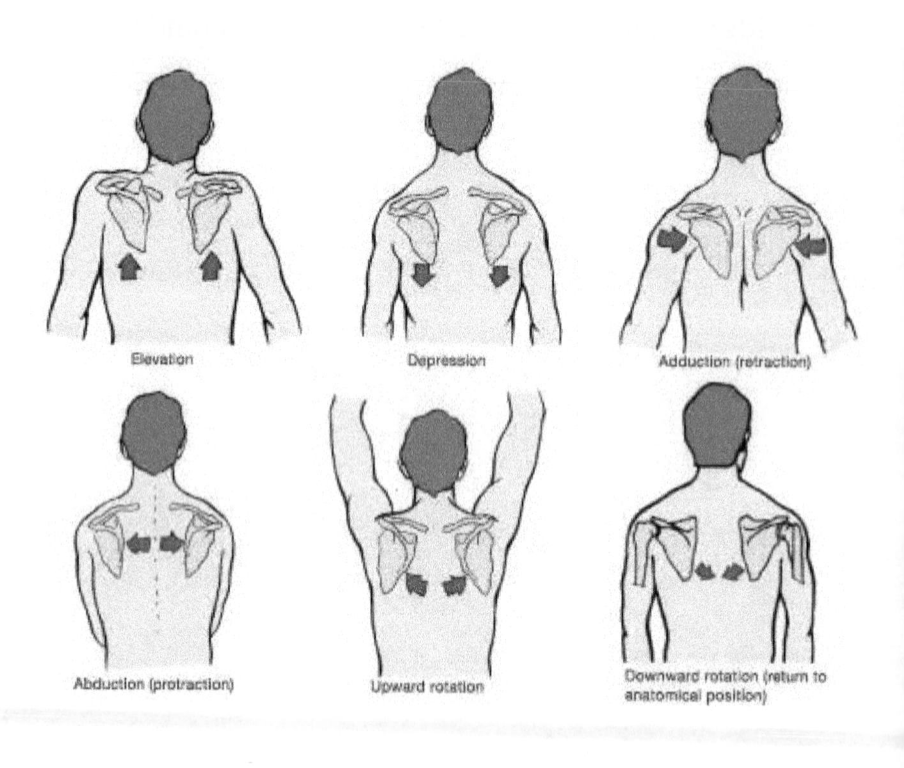

Chapter 2) Anatomy of the Shoulder Joint

A joint is the point where two or more bones come into contact with each other. As the human body consists of 206 bones, there are more than 300 joints in a body. The shoulder joint is one of the most important, major joints of the body.

The shoulder joint falls under the category of diarthrosis joints, which are freely movable joints. The shoulder is the most mobile joint of the human body. The bones that contribute to form the shoulder joint are connected by an articular capsule, which is surrounded by ligaments. Hence the shoulder joint is considered a synovial joint.

There are 3 joints in the shoulder region.

1. Glenohumeral joint (the "actual" shoulder joint)

2. Acromioclavicular joint

3. Sternoclavicular joint

The Glenohumeral joint is the actual shoulder joint, which is attached to the main skeletal system, or spine, by acromioclavicular and sternoclavicular joints.

Like any other joint, the shoulder joint (glenohumeral joint) also has components of its own.

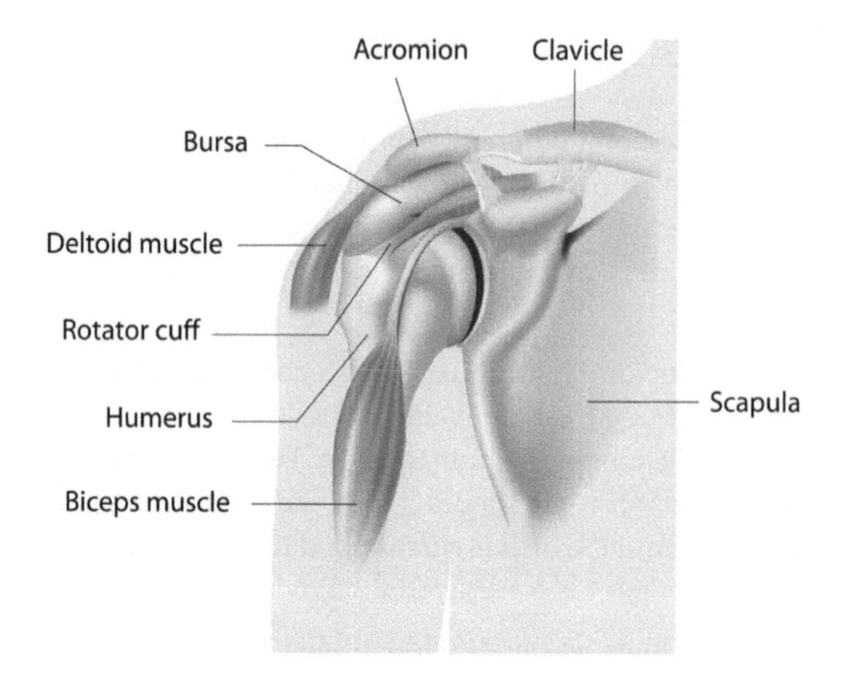

1) Bones & Articular Surfaces:

The bony components of shoulder joint are:

- Head of the Humerus (upper arm bone)

- Glenoid fossa of the Scapula (shoulder blade bone)

Humeral head represents a ball where glenoid fossa represents a socket; hence this is classified as a synovial joint of "ball and socket" variety.

In addition to this articulation, the scapula connects with the clavicle (collar bone) forming the acromioclavicular joint, whereas the clavicle connects with the sternum (breast bone) forming the sternoclavicular joint. Because of these two joints, the upper limbs of a human body link up with the main vertical skeletal system.

2) Muscles & Tendons:

As the shoulder is considered the most mobile joint of the body, the muscles surrounding the shoulder have to be large and powerful to perform strong movements. The shallow "socket" of the scapula promotes the mobility of the joint, in spite of the fact that it increases the risk of misplacing or slipping of the humeral head during forceful movements of the shoulder. This is prevented by a protective muscular cuff named as "rotator cuff".

The rotator cuff is formed up of 4 muscles.

- Supraspinatus
- Subscapularis
- Infraspinatus
- Teres minor

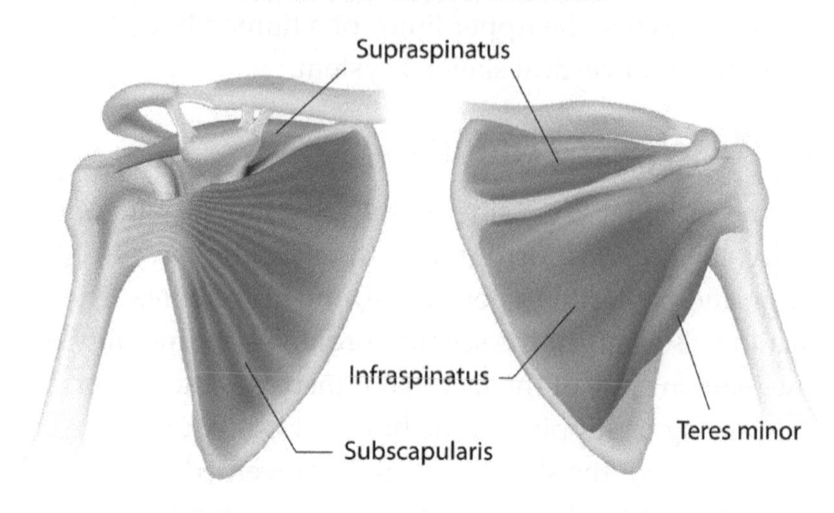

In addition to the rotator cuff muscles, the following muscles contribute to the powerful movements of the shoulder:

- Deltoid
- Pectoralis major
- Latissimus dorsi

Besides, Teres major also contributes to the movements of the shoulder joint.

Any muscle in the human body attaches to a bone/s. This attachment is done via a thick, fibrous connective tissue called tendon. Tendons and muscles work collaboratively.

As a tendon transmits the force generated by a muscle, tendons are also prone to injuries.

The following table contains the attachments, nerve supply and the actions of the musculature of the shoulder joint. Additional features are also tabulated.

Attachments	Nerve supply	Movements	Additional points
Supraspinatus			
Originating from the Upper part of the back of the scapula (Supraspinous fossa) Inserting into the Outer part of the upper end of the humeral head (greater tubercle)	Suprascapular nerve (C5, C6)	Shoulder abduction– initiating part	- A rotator cuff muscle - Initiator of the sideway movements of arms - Most common muscle/ tendon to get injured
Subscapularis			
Originating from the Inner part of the front of the scapula (Subscapular fossa) Inserting into the Inner upper end of the humeral head (lesser tubercle)	Upper & lower subscapular nerves (C5, C6, C7)	Shoulder medial rotation	- A rotator cuff muscle

Infraspinatus			
Originating from the Lower, inner part of the back of the scapula (Infraspinous fossa) Inserting into the Outer part of upper end of the humeral head (greater tubercle)	Suprascapular nerve (C5, C6)	Shoulder lateral rotation	- A rotator cuff muscle
Teres minor			
Originating from the Upper, outer border of the back of the scapula Inserting into the Outer part of the upper end of the humeral head (greater tubercle)	Auxiliary nerve (C5, C6)	Shoulder lateral rotation	- A rotator cuff muscle

Attachments	Nerve supply	Mvts	Additional points
Latissimus dorsi			
Originating from the Pelvis, thoracic spine, ribs & lowest point of the scapula Inserting into the Outer part of the humerus (Floor of the bicipital groove)	Thoracodorsal nerve (C6, C7, C8)	Shoulder extension Shoulder adduction Shoulder medial rotation	-Helps in activities like swimming, rowing, climbing, pulling etc. -Helps in coughing & sneezing -Holds scapula in situ
Teres major			
Originating from the Lower, outer border of the back of the scapula Inserting into the Outer part of upper end of the humeral head (greater tubercle)	Lower subscapular nerve (C5, C6, C7)	Shoulder extension Shoulder adduction Shoulder medial rotation	-Works along with the Latissimus dorsi

.ttachments	Nerve supply	Myths	Additional points
ectoralis major			
)riginating from the :lavicle, Sternum and artilages of the ribs nserting into theOuter art of the humerus Lateral part of the icipital groove)	Medial & Lateral pectoral nerves (C5, C6, C7, C8, T1)	Shoulder adduction Shoulder medial rotation Shoulder flexion Shoulder extension	-Muscle of the breast -Main muscle that works in pressing the fists against each other (horizontal adduction) -Helps in activities like climbing up
)eltoid			
)riginating from the Outer art of the clavicle and 2 ony prominences of the capula (Lower part of the pine of the scapula and)uter part of the acromion f the scapula) nserting into the Outer part f the humerus (deltoid uberosity)	Auxiliary nerve (C5, C6)	Shoulder flexion Shoulder extension Shoulder abduction Shoulder medial rotation Shoulder lateral rot.	-Most powerful muscle in the shoulder joint -Very important in overhead activities

3) Joint Capsule & Ligaments:

In relation to the skeletal muscles, a ligament is the fibrous band that connects one bone to another, especially in forming joints. Ligaments assist in stabilizing a joint. Sometimes it limits or prevents particular movements of the joint.

The capsule consists of two layers; the outer layer is mainly made of fibrous tissue whereas the inner layer is a secreting layer. The inner layer is named as the synovial membrane. It produces synovial fluid, which helps in lubricating the joint in performing movements. The shoulder capsule is comparatively very thin. The front and lower parts of the capsule are least supported, so that they promote the dislocation of the shoulder. To overcome this, three glenohumeral ligaments have been developed to strengthen the front of the shoulder.

Apart from the capsule, there are several other ligaments available such as coracohumeral, transverse humeral, acromioclavicular and coracoacromial ligaments.

4) Bursae

Bursae are fluid filled sacs that cushion in between bones and tendons and/or muscles.

Bursae that can be seen in the shoulder joint are mentioned below:

- Subdeltoid bursa/ Subacromial bursa

- Subscapular bursa/ Subtendinous bursa of subscapularis muscle

- Infraspinatus bursa

5) Adjacent Nerves

The auxiliary nerve is the main nerve that has close contact with the glenohumeral joint, as it winds up around the neck of the humerus.

There is a risk of damaging the nerve during dislocations of the shoulder.

Chapter 3) Problems Associated With the Shoulder Joint

There can be numerous problems affecting one or more components of the shoulder joint. Some of them are mentioned below:

1) *Instability & Dislocations*

As the "socket" of the shoulder joint is very shallow, the humeral head is more prone to slip out of the socket. The slipping of the humeral head out of the socket is called as dislocation. The tendency to dislocate the shoulder is known as shoulder instability.

Shoulder dislocation can be partial or complete. Partial dislocation, also termed as "subluxation", means the humeral head partly comes out of the socket. In a complete dislocation, the humeral head completely comes out of the socket.

Dislocation of the shoulder can be of several types; forward (anterior dislocation), backward (posterior dislocation) and downward (inferior dislocation). Anterior dislocation is the most common type of shoulder dislocation.

Shoulder Dislocation

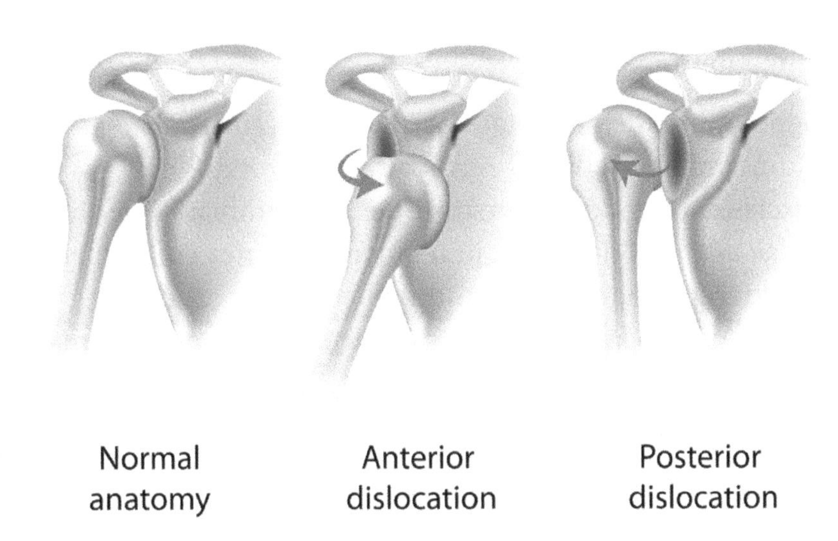

The main reason for shoulder dislocation is severe trauma to the shoulder. In rare cases, especially in people born with ligament laxity, shoulder dislocation can happen due to weak or overstretched ligaments.

The main symptoms of shoulder dislocation include swelling, bruising, numbness and weakness.

A dislocated shoulder without rehabilitation promotes episodes of recurrent dislocations. This chronic shoulder instability further weakens the capsule and other ligaments.

2) Rotator Cuff Injuries

The rotator cuff is the protective muscular cuff surrounding the shoulder joint. As the shoulder is the most mobile joint in the human body with the least protective mechanisms, it is more viable to injuries. Especially the muscles and tendons of the rotator cuff, which act towards the protection of the shoulder joint, are at a higher risk of getting injured.

These injuries can be rotator cuff tears, strains, and tendinopathies, which directly affect the rotator cuff muscles and tendons. Bursitis due to inflammation of the bursae also could be seen in relation to rotator cuff injuries. Shoulder impingement syndrome is another condition where muscles and tendons of the rotator cuff get inflamed and irritated. Less attention to management of these injuries may lead to a frozen shoulder.

These conditions are to be discussed in detail in subsequent chapters of the book.

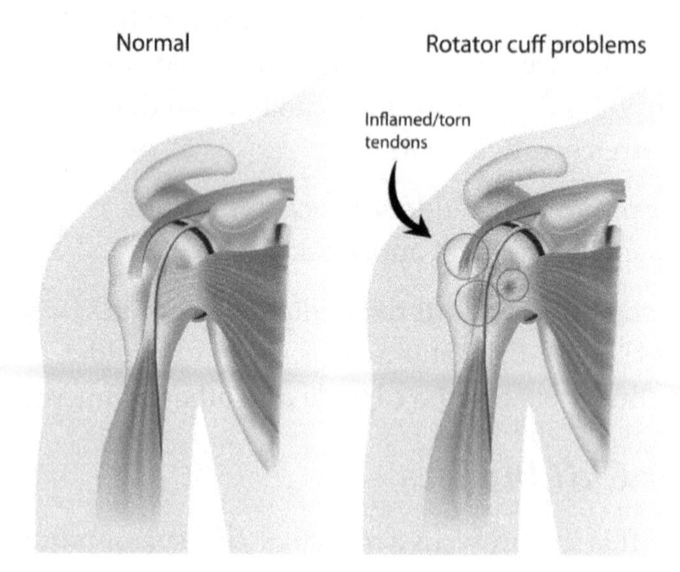

3) Ligament Injuries

Ligaments hold the upper arm bone, shoulder blade and the collarbone in appropriate places to form the shoulder and acromioclavicular joints. Injuries to these ligaments may lead to the disjointing of the associated bones, hence it is called separation.

In most cases, the acromioclavicular ligament is getting injured, causing the separation of the acromioclavicular joint.

A ligament injury can be mild (Grade I), moderate (Grade II) or severe (Grade III). Mild acromioclavicular separation is a minor sprain to the ligament. Moderate acromioclavicular separation engages with a tear of the acromioclavicular ligament and a minor sprain of the costoclavicular ligament. Severe injury implicates a tear of both the acromioclavicular and costoclavicular ligaments.

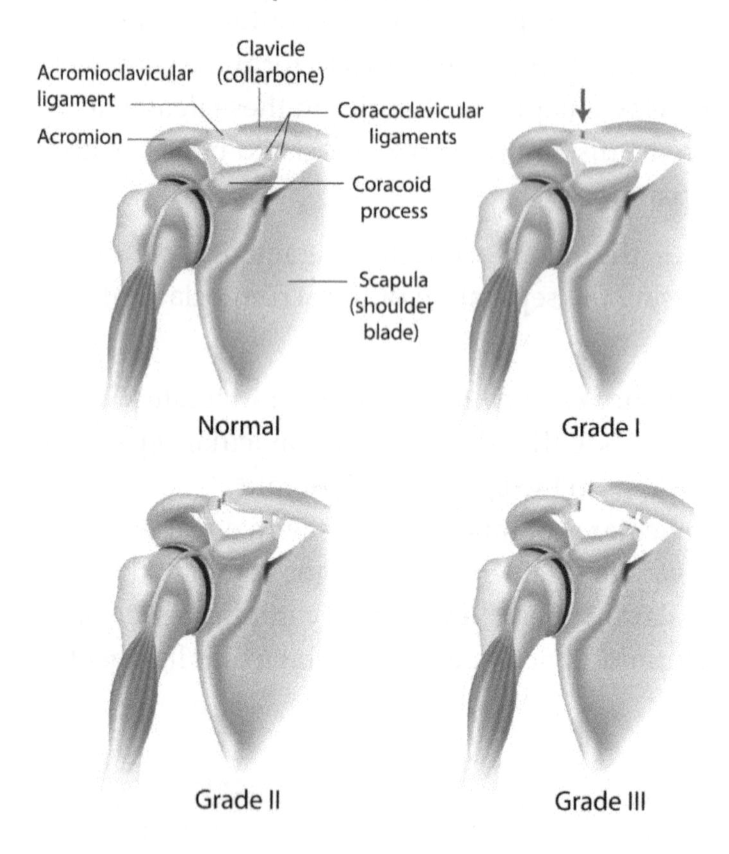

The most common cause of the injury is falling directly on the shoulder. Other causes include skate boarding, rowing, combat sports such as boxing, judo and Muay Thai in addition to contact sports such as football, rugby and wrestling.

The most common symptoms of ligament injury are pain (ranging from mild to severe depending on the grade of the injury), tenderness of the shoulder, bruising and swelling. The range of the shoulder movements has been reduced. Weakness of the shoulder and arm muscles is evident if untreated properly over a long period of time. In more severe injuries, a bump can be seen on the shoulder, which indicates a complete separation with/ without displacement of the collarbone and upper arm bone.

Shoulder separation can be treated surgically or conservatively.

Chapter 4) Acute Management of a Musculoskeletal Injury

Within the first few days of the injury, "PRICER" is the best treatment protocol for any muscle tear.

It is compulsory to refrain from using the "HARM" protocol in the acute phase. HARM aggravates the blood leakage out of the vessels.

1) "PRICER" Protocol

P: Protection

Protection is to prevent further damage to the area. For example, if you were carrying a heavy weight when you hear the snapping sound of the shoulder, you must hold off the weight immediately.

R: Rest

The affected area should not be mobilized in any means at the onset of the injury. Movements might promote further injury to the site.

Various appliances can be used to prevent movements. The sling is the most common, simple technique of promoting rest in rotator cuff tears. In addition, casts and splints also can be used.

I: Ice

Ice or cold therapy plays a main role in acute management of a muscle tear. In an acute injury, muscle fibers tear away, meanwhile tiny blood vessels within the muscle also may get ruptured. Bleeding within the muscle may increase swelling and pain. Cold therapy helps in shrinking these ruptured blood vessels, resulting in less bleeding.

It is advisable to apply ice/ cold therapy for the first 2-3 days (48-72 hours), for 20 minutes duration in 2 hourly intervals.

C: Compression

Compression assists in reducing the swelling. Additional pressure applied during compression constricts the blood vessels, hence preventing swelling.

Bandaging and using compression material such as Tubigrips is the best way of managing swelling.

E: Elevation

The injured body part should be elevated above the level of the heart. As the shoulder is naturally situated above the level of the heart, elevation is automatically achieved.

R: Referral

An injury should be treated by a healthcare professional. A General Practitioner will inform you about further management needed and refer you to an orthopaedic surgeon, a physiotherapist or an occupational therapist for further management.

2) "HARM" Protocol

H: Heat

In the first 2-3 days of the musculoskeletal injury, heating up of the area should be avoided. Heat promotes vasodilatation, causing an increase in blood leakage. Heat also enhances the inflammatory process, therefore aggravates the condition. Swelling occurs due to these factors.

A: Alcohol

Alcohol promotes the permeability of blood vessels. Hence, it increases the blood leakage out of the vessels. Consuming alcohol will increase the risk of swelling and bruising.

R: Running

Running, in HARM, is not the vocabulary meaning. Running in this protocol means the activities. Most of the time, the first thing you do after an injury is to see whether the joint/ body part can be moved or not. This promotes further damage. Hence, any planned activity should be avoided in the acute phase.

M: Massage

The most common reaction of people during an injury is massage, in other words – rubbing. This is an improper practice, which leads to an increase in the local temperature of the area. An increase in the temperature induces the inflammatory reaction of the affected area.

For the first 2-3 days of the onset of the injury, ice is the best treatment. After 3 days, instead of cold therapy, heat therapy can be used. Hot packs, Infra-Red Therapy and heating pads can be used for this purpose. It enhances the blood supply to the area, so that the chemical substances that cause pain are washed away with the blood flow.

Chapter 5) General Treatment Strategies of a Chronic Musculoskeletal Injury

Treatment strategies for chronic musculoskeletal injuries are under 2 main management categories: pharmacological and non-pharmacological management.

1) Pharmacological Management

Medications reduce the inflammatory reaction and therefore reduce the pain. Analgesics, in common terms – painkillers, are the drugs used to relieve pain. Topical analgesics, Paracetamol, Non Steroidal Anti Inflammatory Drugs (NSAIDs), local anaesthetics and corticosteroids are the main drug types used in musculoskeletal injuries.

a) Topical Analgesics

Topical analgesics are the analgesics that work on the nerves of the peripheries. They are usually applied over the skin as a gel. It is the best option for people who are having systemic side effects rather than taking these medications orally.

A few examples for the topical analgesics are stated below:

- Ibuprofen

- Diclofenac

- Capsaicin

b) Paracetamol (Acetaminophen)

Paracetamol is an over-the-counter analgesic and an antipyretic drug. It has very few side effects. Yet, overdose and prolonged usage of Paracetamol may lead to liver damage and kidney damage.

c) Non Steroidal Anti Inflammatory Drugs (NSAIDs)

NSAIDs reduce the pain; meanwhile lessening the degree of inflammation of the muscles and tendons. They have side effects such as peptic ulcers, kidney failure and allergic reactions.

Aspirin, Naproxen and Ibuprofen are the most commonly used NSAIDs worldwide.

d) Local Anesthetics and Corticosteroids

These are given as local injections intramuscularly. This is the ultimate option that can be chosen to alleviate pain.

2) Non-Pharmacological Management

Physiotherapy is the most common type of non-pharmacological management in musculoskeletal injuries. Physiotherapy management is important as it enhances the rate of healing and ensures the functional independence of the patient. Several treatment strategies are included in this management.

a) Heat Therapy

Heat Therapy is to treat injuries using heat. There are numerous mechanisms of applying heat.

Heat can be either moist or dry. A homemade hot pack is an example of moist heat, whereas Infra Red (IR) therapy is an example of dry heat. Moist heat penetrates the skin more than dry heat.

Heat can also be either superficial or deep. Hot packs, heating pads, and IR give a superficial heat. Short Wave Diathermy (SWD) and Ultra Sound Therapy (UST) give a deep localized heat.

b) Soft Tissue Massage

This is appropriate only for partial tears at the chronic stage. Massage techniques for the incomplete tears mainly include friction and kneading.

Friction:

Friction is a deep manipulative technique performed over a precise anatomical structure occupying a small area by thumbs or fingers. The adhesions formed in the deeper levels after minor tears of a muscle/ tendon are deformed via friction.

There are 2 techniques of friction; circular and transverse. Circular friction is suitable for a muscle tear, whereas transverse friction is suitable for a tendon rupture.

Kneading:

Kneading is to move the skin and subcutaneous tissue in a circular motion over the underlying tissues. It helps to increase the blood and lymphatic flow to the area while breaking down the adhesions formed in the subcutaneous tissues, therefore reducing the pain. This can be performed with the palm, fingers, thumbs, 1-2 finger/s or elbows.

c) Electrotherapy

The best electrotherapy practice is Ultra-Sound Therapy (UST). Therapeutic ultrasound waves are used for treatment purposes. They are transmitted into the body via a transducer placed on the skin. A therapeutic gel is used as a coupling medium to transmit the ultrasound wave effectively in to the body.

The frequency is set according to the depth of the affected tissue and the mode is set according to the onset of the injury. As rotator cuff muscles are superficial, that is, not deeper than 2cm, the frequency can be set at 3MHz. When considering the mode, continuous mode is effective in chronic conditions, whereas pulse mode is beneficial in acute conditions.

The treatment duration varies according to the size of the affected tissue. Usually an area of $10cm^2$ is treated for 1-2 minutes. Thrice a week is the ideal number of sessions.

Apart from UST, Transcutaneous Electrical Nerve Stimulator (TENS) can also be used to alleviate pain.

d) Physical Exercises

Physical exercises play a main role in the rehabilitation phase of any musculoskeletal injury.

Physical exercises can be categorized as stretching, strengthening and mobilization exercises.

These exercise types are discussed in detail in the chapter after the following chapter (Chapter 7).

e) Postural Awareness

Most musculoskeletal pains are due to mechanical problems. A muscle imbalance results in posture variances. These postural defects are a causative factor for muscle pains. Hence postural awareness and postural correction is very essential in a treatment procedure.

Chapter 6) Getting Ready for the Exercises

Most people think that exercises can be performed by anyone at anytime, anywhere for any duration. Most times they search for some exercises, probably on the Internet, TV or a magazine, and perform them as it is. For example, if a woman has excessive abdominal fat, she may look up fat burning exercises on the Internet and perform them. She might have physical limitations when performing exercises or some medical condition that means she has to be very cautious when performing exercises. In some circumstances, it is not the fat burning that needs to be addressed, but a separate root cause for accumulating fat in the tissues beneath the skin of the abdomen. Therefore it is advisable to seek for proper medical advice that is appropriate for ones' self when performing exercises.

1) "FITT" principle

Physical exercises cannot be performed as a one off. FITT principle allows you to find the proper training program with the correct timing.

a) F: Frequency

This is the number of times you perform exercises. If you are a novice, start from low frequency and go up to high frequency. For an example, start with 3 times per week and proceed to 5-6 times per week.

b) I: Intensity

This is the level of effort you exert in exercises. In other words, it is the number of repetitions you perform per exercise session. For example, stretching has to be performed with 10 repetitions whereas strength exercises have to be performed with 30 repetitions.

c) T: Type

The type of exercise you perform falls under this category. It might be strength training or aerobics.

d) T: Time

The duration of the exercise is termed as 'Time'. For example, when performing stretching it takes at least 1 minute to perform 1 stretch properly. Therefore the total duration would be 10 minutes if there were 10 repetitions.

2) Factors to consider when planning an exercise program

a) Goal of the exercise program

You should set a proper goal for your exercise program. The goal you set should be "SMART".

S: Specific (targeting some specific area. E.g.: strengthening, aerobics etc.)

M: Measurable (stating an indicator of progress. E.g.: ROM of joints, grade of movement, amount of body weight etc.)

A: Attainable (considering the ability to achieve. E.g.: achieving 50% of pain relief within next 2 sessions)

R: Realistic (stating realistic goals. E.g.: reducing the body weight by 10kg in a week is impossible)

T: Time-bound (stating the time duration. E.g.: performing the exercise with XX repetitions XX times XX days per week)

b) Age

The exercise intensity and severity of exercise and exercise platforms differ according to your age. For example; bar hanging is ideal for an 18-year old male, but not for a 70-year old male. Age is a non-modifiable factor.

c) Gender

Exercise protocols for men are mostly different to women's. Gender is also a non-modifiable factor.

d) Medical history

You should be cautious if you have high blood pressure, cardiovascular diseases, diabetes and respiratory diseases such as asthma.

e) Adequate nutrition

You should have a balanced diet in all cases. Adequate water intake during the exercises is very essential.

3) Warm-up Session

a) Objective

Prepare the muscles for the exercise procedure by increasing flexibility and adequate blood supply to the area.

b) Time Duration

10 – 15 minutes prior to exercising.

c) Constituents

5 – 10 minutes jogging with arm movements (arm rotation, forearm rotation, shoulder rotation etc.) – to increase body temperature.

10 – 15 minutes stretching of the shoulder muscles – to increase flexibility.

d) Benefits of warm-up

- Keep elasticity of the muscles
- Increase the range of motion of joints
- Increase flexibility
- Enhance coordination of vision, joint position and muscles
- Increase heart rate and body temperature
- Increase blood flow to muscles
- Prevent injuries

4) Cool-down Session

a) Objective

Normalize bodily functions.

b) Time Duration

10 – 15 minutes after exercising.

c) Constituents

5 – 10 minutes jogging with arm movements (arm rotation, forearm rotation, shoulder rotation etc.) – to decrease body temperature and eliminate waste products.

10 – 15 minutes stretching of the shoulder muscles – to normalize the muscle tone.

d) Benefits of cool-down

- Obtain a gradual decrease of the heart rate and blood pressure rate to resting or pre-exercise levels

- Normalize the respiratory rate

5) Injury Prevention

a) "PRICER" Protocol

Refer Chapter 4.

b) Kinesio Taping

Kinesio taping helps in preventing the unnecessary movements of the shoulder. Hence it is a preventive mechanism as well as a treatment technique.

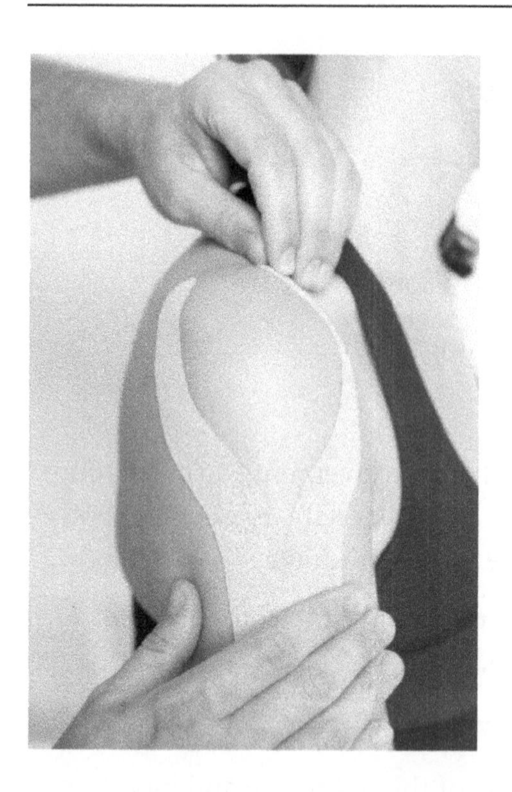

Kinesio taping for rotator cuff tear:

Placing Anchors:

- Keep the hand on same side hip.

- Place a strip of tape around the upper arm, keeping the biceps tense.

- Place another strip of tape from the shoulder blade to the chest.

- Remember, these should be applied gently to prevent circulatory problems.

Straight Lines:

- Keep the hand on same side hip.

- Start the tape at the level of the upper arm anchor at the side of the arm.

- Do 1 – 3 straight lines depending on the amount of support required, with each additional line partially overlapping the previous line.

Shoulder Crosses:

- Keep the hand on same side hip.

- Start the tape at the level of the upper arm anchor at the front of the arm and go up to the back of the shoulder blade-chest anchor.

- Two lines of tape should be used, forming a cross.

- Do 1-2 crosses depending on the amount of support required.

- Close the anchors by applying a sealing tape.

Chapter 7) Physical Exercises Performed in Rotator Cuff Injuries

Physical exercise is the main component of rehabilitation in any musculoskeletal injury.

They can be categorized into 3 main categories; mobilization, stretching and strengthening exercises.

1) Shoulder Mobilization Exercises

Shoulder mobilization exercises help in increasing the range of motion of the shoulder. Shoulder mobilization has to be done in every movement direction of the shoulder.

Remember:

Do not go beyond your normal range of the shoulder.

Do not hold your breath.

Be cautious about pain. Do not perform if the pain increases.

a) Increase Flexion

ROM Fl Exe 1:

Sit upright in front of a table. Slide your forearm forwards along the table as you bend from the waist until a stretch is felt. Come back to the starting position.

Repeat 10 times. Do 3 sessions per day.

ROM Fl Exe 2:

Stand with a broomstick/wand holding it with two hands. Lift forward the maximum you can. Come back to the starting position.

Repeat 10 times. Do 3 sessions per day.

b) Increase Extension

ROM Ext Exe 1:

Stand turning your back to a table. Keep feet shoulder-width apart. Hold the table with both hands. Gently lower body by bending knees until stretch is felt at the front of the shoulder. Come back to the starting position.

Repeat 10 times. Do 3 sessions per day.

ROM Ext Exe 2:

Lie down facing downward. Hold a broomstick/wand with two hands behind your back. Lift backwards from the buttocks until a stretch is felt at the shoulder. Come back to the starting position.

Repeat 10 times. Do 3 sessions per day.

c) Increase Abduction

ROM Abd Exe 1:

Stand upright. Bring arms straight out to side and raise as high as possible without pain. Slowly come down to the starting position.

Repeat 10 times. Do 3 sessions per day.

ROM Abd Exe 2:

Stand upright. Hold the wand with the affected side palm up and unaffected side palm down. Push wand directly out from your side with unaffected hand until you feel a stretch at the shoulder. Come back to the starting position.

Repeat 10 times. Do 3 sessions per day.

d) Increase External Rotation

ROM ER Exe 1:

Stand parallel to a doorframe. Keep palm of hand against the doorframe and elbow bent at 90^{0}. Turn your body towards your unaffected side with the hand against the doorframe and elbow at 90^{0} until a stretch is felt at the shoulder. Return to the starting position.

Repeat 10 times. Do 3 sessions per day.

ROM ER Exe 2:

Stand upright. Hold wand with affected side palm up and unaffected side palm down. Keep elbows bent and tuck to your body. Push with unaffected side out from body while keeping elbow at side until you feel a stretch at the shoulder. Be sure to keep elbows bent. Come back to the starting position.

Repeat 10 times. Do 3 sessions per day.

e) Increase Internal Rotation

ROM IR Exe 1:

Stand upright. Hold wand with affected side palm up and unaffected side palm down. Keep elbows bent and tuck to your body. Pull with unaffected side across the body while keeping elbow at side until you feel a stretch at the shoulder. Be sure to keep elbows bent. Come back to the starting position.

Repeat 10 times. Do 3 sessions per day.

ROM IR Exe 2:

Stand upright. Hold a towel behind the back. Pull affected arm up behind back by pulling towel upward with unaffected arm. Come back to the starting position.

Repeat 10 times. Do 3 sessions per day.

f) Increase Horizontal Abduction/ Adduction

ROM HAbd/HAdd Exe 1:

Stand upright. Hold a wand, keeping both palms down. Push wand across body with unaffected side. Then pull back across body, keeping the arm parallel to the floor. Do not allow your trunk to twist.

Repeat 10 times. Do 3 sessions per day.

g) Increase Overall Mobility (Codman's Exercises)

ROM Codman Exe 1:

Bend forward holding a table. Let arm move in a circle clockwise, then counterclockwise by rocking body weight in a circular pattern.

Repeat 20 times. Do 3 sessions per day.

ROM Codman Exe 2:

Bend forward holding a table. Gently move arm from side to side by rocking body weight from side to side. Let arm swing freely.

Repeat 20 times. Do 3 sessions per day.

ROM Codman Exe 3:

Bend forward towards a table. Hold the table with unaffected hand and support body weight. Reach across body as far as you can, then pull back.

Repeat 20 times. Do 3 sessions per day.

2) Shoulder Stretching Exercises

Stretching has to be performed in correct methodology.

Slowly perform the movement until you feel a mild stretch. Hold on in that position for 30 seconds. Then further stretch the shoulder. Hold for 30 seconds. Ease.

Remember:

Do not bounce back and forth in the procedure of stretching.

Do not hold your breath.

Be cautious about pain. Do not perform if the pain increases.

a) Stretch Shoulder Flexors (at the front of the shoulder)

Stretch Fl Exe 1:

Stand turning your back to a table. Keep feet shoulder-width apart. Hold the table with both hands. Gently lower your body by bending your knees until stretch is felt at the front of the shoulder. Hold for 30 seconds. Come back to the starting position.

Repeat 10 times. Do 3 sessions per day.

b) Stretch Shoulder Extensors (at back of the shoulder)

Stretch Ext Exe 1:

Sit upright in front of a table. Slide forearm forward along the table as you bend from the waist until a stretch is felt. Hold for 30 seconds. Come back to the starting position.

Repeat 10 times. Do 3 sessions per day.

c) Stretch Shoulder Adductors (at armpit) & Horizontal Adductors (at chest)

Stretch Add/HAdd Exe 1:

Stand facing a wall and place your affected arm against it at 90^0 from the shoulder. Keep your shoulder and arm flat against the wall. Rotate your body outwards by moving your feet. When you feel a stretch along your chest, hold for about 30 seconds. If you are comfortable with the stretch felt with your body perpendicular to the wall, move your arm upwards to further stretch and repeat the procedure.

Repeat 10 times. Do 3 sessions per day.

Stretch Add/HAdd Exe 2:

Stand at a corner of a wall. Place your forearms on the perpendicular walls making a 90^0 angle at the shoulder. Move your trunk towards the corner of the wall. When you feel a stretch along your chest, hold for about 30 seconds. If you are comfortable with the stretch felt, move your forearms slightly up to further stretch and repeat the procedure.

Repeat 10 times. Do 3 sessions per day.

d) Stretch Shoulder Internal Rotators

Stretch IR Exe 1:

Stand parallel to a doorframe. Keep palm of hand against doorframe and elbow bent at 90^0. Turn body towards your unaffected side with the hand against doorframe and elbow at 90^0, until a stretch is felt at the shoulder. Hold for 30 seconds. Return to the starting position.

Repeat 10 times. Do 3 sessions per day.

Stretch IR Exe 2:

Stand upright. Hold wand with affected side palm up and unaffected side palm down. Keep elbows bent and tuck to your body. Push with unaffected side out from body while keeping elbow at side until you feel a stretch at the shoulder. Be sure to keep elbows bent. Hold for about 30 seconds. Come back to the starting position.

Repeat 10 times. Do 3 sessions per day.

e) Stretch Shoulder External Rotators

Stretch ER Exe 1:

Stand upright. Hold wand with affected side palm up and unaffected side palm down. Keep elbows bent and tuck to your body. Pull with unaffected hand across the body while keeping your elbow at your side until you feel a stretch at the shoulder. Be sure to keep elbows bent. Hold for about 30 seconds. Come back to the starting position.

Repeat 10 times. Do 3 sessions per day.

Stretch ER Exe 2:

Stand upright. Hold a towel behind your back. Pull affected arm up behind the back by pulling the towel upwards with the unaffected arm. Hold for about 30 seconds. Come back to the starting position.

Repeat 10 times. Do 3 sessions per day.

f) Stretch Shoulder Joint Capsule

Stretch Capsule Exe 1:

Stand/sit upright. Raise your arm forward 90^0 while keeping the elbow bent. Gently pull on the elbow with the opposite hand until a stretch is felt in the back of the shoulder. Hold for about 30 seconds. Ease. This process stretches the posterior part (back) of the capsule.

Repeat 10 times. Do 3 sessions per day.

Stretch Capsule Exe 2:

Stand/sit upright. Raise your arm sideways with the elbow bent. Gently pull on elbow with opposite hand until a stretch is felt in the armpit. Hold for about 30 seconds. Come back to the starting position. This process stretches the inferior part (lower part) of the capsule.

Repeat 10 times. Do 3 sessions per day.

3) Shoulder Strengthening Exercises

Strengthening is the most important part in the rehabilitation phase. The weight used in strengthening differs from person to person. Therefore you have to choose the appropriate weight for you. Let us assume that you lift a particular amount of weight, for example 500g. You feel no pain or difficulty in lifting that amount of weight. Then you have to try a weight of 600g. If that is also workable with you, add another 100g and then another 100g etc. Let us assume that you felt a very slight pain when you lifted 800g. Add more 100g and see whether it is tolerable. If you can't lift it at all, then the weight appropriate for you is 800g. If you feel a mild pain though you can perform the movement, use 900g as the appropriate weight for you. The usual recommendation is 10 repetitions per 1 session.

a) Strengthening Shoulder Flexors

Strength Fl Exe 1:

Stand upright. Keep feet shoulder-width apart. Take the appropriate weight for you as described earlier. Lift the weight forward and upward as slowly as you can, through your pain free range of motion. Come back to the starting position.

Repeat with 3 sets of 10 repetitions.

Strength Fl Exe 2:

Stand upright. Take a tube/resistive band and tie it onto the floor. Using tubing, start with your arm at your side and pull the arm forward and upward as slowly as you can. Move shoulder through pain free range of motion. Come back to the starting position.

Repeat with 3 sets of 10 repetitions.

b) Strengthening Shoulder Extensors

Strength Ext Exe 1:

Stand upright against a wall. Press the back of the arm into the wall using light resistance. Hold for 10 seconds and release. Progress into moderate and maximal resistances.

Repeat with 3 sets of 10 repetitions.

Strength Ext Exe 2:

Stand upright. Keep feet shoulder-width apart. Take the appropriate weight for you as described earlier. Lift the weight outward and backward as slowly as you can, through your pain free range of motion. Come back to the starting position.

Repeat with 3 sets of 10 repetitions.

Strength Ext Exe 3:

Stand upright. Take a tube/resistive band and tie it to the floor. Using tubing, start with your arm at your side and pull the arm outward and backward as slowly as you can. Move the shoulder through pain free range of motion. Come back to the starting position.

Repeat with 3 sets of 10 repetitions.

c) Strengthening Shoulder Abductors

Strength Abd Exe 1:

Stand upright facing parallel to a wall. Make sure your affected shoulder is at the side of the wall. Press the side of your arm into the wall using light resistance. Hold for 10 seconds and release. Progress into moderate and maximal resistances.

Repeat with 3 sets of 10 repetitions.

Strength Abd Exe 2:

Stand upright. Keep feet shoulder-width apart. Take the appropriate weight for you as described earlier. Lift the weight sideways as slowly as you can, through your pain free range of motion. Come back to the starting position.

Repeat with 3 sets of 10 repetitions.

Strength Abd Exe 3:

Stand upright. Take a tube/resistive band and tie it to the floor. Using tubing, start with the arm at your side and pull the arm upward sideways as slowly as you can. Move shoulder through pain free range of motion. Come back to the starting position.

Repeat with 3 sets of 10 repetitions.

d) Strengthening Shoulder Internal Rotators

Strength IR Exe 1:

Attach the tube/resistive band to a wall parallel to your elbow level when sitting. Sit upright on the chair with the affected shoulder facing the wall. Using tubing, and keeping the elbow in at the side, rotate arm inward across the body. Be sure to keep forearm parallel to floor.

Repeat with 3 sets of 10 repetitions.

e) Strengthening Shoulder External Rotators

Strength ER Exe 1:

Lie on your unaffected side (lower arm). Take the appropriate weight for you with the affected side (upper arm). Bring arm upward from the body, keeping the elbow bent and tucked to the trunk.

Repeat with 3 sets of 10 repetitions.

Strength ER Exe 2:

Attach the tube/resistive band to a wall parallel to your elbow level when sitting. Sit upright on the chair, unaffected shoulder facing the wall. Using tubing, and keeping the elbow tucked to the trunk, rotate affected arm outward out of the body. Be sure to keep forearm parallel to the floor.

Repeat with 3 sets of 10 repetitions.

f) Strengthening Shoulder Horizontal Abductors

Strength HAbd Exe 1:

Sit or stand with feet shoulder-width apart and tubing or resistive band looped around each hand. With arms straight out in front, stretch tubing across chest.

Repeat with 3 sets of 10 repetitions.

Strength HAbd Exe 2:

Stand against a doorframe. Raise the arm to 90^0 sideways. Using the doorframe to provide resistance, press the outside of the arm into frame using light resistance. Hold for 10 seconds and release. Progress into moderate and maximal resistances. Make sure you keep upper arm parallel to floor and elbow bent to 90^0.

Repeat with 3 sets of 10 repetitions.

g) Strengthening Shoulder Horizontal Adductors

Strength HAdd Exe 1:

Stand beside a doorframe. Raise the arm to 90^0 sideways. Use the doorframe to provide resistance. Press inner aspect of elbow into the frame giving light resistance. Hold for 10 seconds and release. Progress the exercise with moderate and maximal resistances. Make sure you keep the upper arm parallel to the floor and the elbow bent to 90^0.

Repeat with 3 sets of 10 repetitions.

h) Strengthening Functional Patterns

Strength Function Exe 1:

Attach the tube/resistive band to a wall behind you at your hand level. Quarter turn with the affected side towards the band. Using tubing, pull the affected hand across your body while pushing out with the same arm. This motion is identical to tennis forehand.

Repeat with 3 sets of 10 repetitions.

Strength Function Exe 2:

Attach the tube/resistive band to a wall behind you at your hand level. Quarter turn with the unaffected side towards the band. With feet perpendicular to the tubing and the arm across the body toward tubing attachment, pull across body. This motion is identical to backhand.

Repeat with 3 sets of 10 repetitions.

Strength Function Exe 3:

Attach the tube/resistive band to a wall behind you at your shoulder level. Turn your back to the wall. Pull tubing across body with your affected hand. This motion is identical to serving in tennis or throwing a ball.

Repeat with 3 sets of 10 repetitions.

4) Scapular Stabilization

Scap Stabilize Exe 1:

Sit upright. Keep arms out from sides and elbows bent. Pinch or squeeze shoulder blades together. Hold exercise for 10 seconds. Ease.

Repeat 10 times. Do 3 sessions per day.

Scap Stabilize Exe 2:

Sit upright. Shrug the shoulders. Hold exercise for 10 seconds. Ease.

Repeat 10 times. Do 3 sessions per day.

Scap Stabilize Exe 3:

Sit upright. Bring affected arm across in front of the body. Hold elbow with unaffected arm. Gently pull across chest until a stretch is felt in the back of shoulder. Hold exercise for 10 seconds. Ease. Better to repeat vice versa.

Do 3 sets of 10 reps with 1 minute rest in between sets. Perform in every other day.

Scap Stabilize Exe 4:

Lie facing down. Take your appropriate weight into hands. Bring weight in line with shoulder level (90^0). Keep elbows straight. Raise both arms off of floor. Slowly come back.

Do 3 sets of 10 reps with 1-minute rest in between sets. Perform every other day.

Scap Stabilize Exe 5:

Lie on back. Take your appropriate weight into hands. Bring the arms forward 90^0 (directly over the shoulder joint). Your elbows should be straight. This is your starting position. Move arms up toward ceiling. Return to starting position.

Do 3 sets of 10 reps with a 1-minute rest in between sets. Perform every other day.

Scap Stabilize Exe 6:

Stand with feet shoulder-width apart. Take your appropriate weight into bent hands, palms forward. Now the weight should be at your shoulder level. Raise arms straight up over your head and out to the side.

Do 3 sets of 10 reps with a 1-minute rest in between sets. Perform every other day.

Scap Stabilize Exe 7:

Sit on a chair. Place hands on the seat of the chair. Push down and lift body upward. Lower and repeat.

Do 3 sets of 10 reps with a 1-minute rest in between sets. Perform every other day.

Chapter 8) Rotator Cuff Tear

A muscle is a structure that is made out of long cylindrical fibers that have a contracting and relaxing ability. A muscle tear denotes a break off of these muscle fibers, resulting in poor contractility. A tear sometimes refers to the damage of the tendons that connect the muscles to bones.

Any of the four rotator cuff muscles or their tendons can be torn. It is evident that the Supraspinatus muscle and tendon has the highest possibility of getting injured. Nevertheless, other rotator cuff muscles may also have the risk of getting tears in various circumstances.

A tear can be of two types: partial and complete.

In a partial tear, a few muscle fibers or a part of the tendon are involved. It does not cause a complete separation of the muscle/tendon from the bone; therefore the contracting ability is preserved.

A complete tear, also known as full-thickness tear, fully splits the muscle/tendon. The contracting ability is much more disturbed in a complete tear.

A rotator cuff tear is quite common all over the world regardless of ethnicity, race or geographical variance. There has been a lot of research carried out on this topic.

Recent statistics show that nearly 7.6% of healthy Norwegians aged 50 – 79 years old have a full thickness rotator cuff tear, though they do not notice it. More than 50% of the US patient population older than 65 experience rotator cuff tears. 0.95% of the UK population is suffering from shoulder pain where 85% of them had pain due to rotator cuff tears or tendinopathies.

Evidence shows that rotator cuff tears are directly associated with age.

1) Causes & Risk Factors

Trauma and degeneration are the two main causes for rotator cuff injuries.

Trauma can be due to:

- A sudden thrust on the arm/shoulder (e.g.: falling on your shoulder, using the arm to hang on and prevent falling)

- A sudden force derived from the shoulder muscles (e.g.: lifting a heavy weight)

- Vigorous overhead activities (e.g.: throwing a ball or a javelin)

- Repetitive activities of the shoulder (e.g.: painting, carpentering)

- Certain sports (e.g.: baseball, tennis, badminton, squash, cricket etc.)

Degenerative changes mainly occur due to the ageing process. The blood supply to the muscles may deteriorate. The strength and the quality of the muscle fibers may get reduced. Because of these reasons, rotator cuff tears are more prone in the elderly population.

Risk factors of a rotator cuff injury comprise several factors:

- Being more than 40 years old
- Lifting heavy objects
- Being a sportsman (especially baseball, tennis, and cricket players)
- Working in the construction field (especially carpenters, and painters)
- Poor postural adherence (especially rounded shoulders)
- Having weak shoulder muscles (could be due to inactivity or a previous trauma)

2) Signs & Symptoms

a) Pain and Tenderness

The main symptom of rotator cuff tears is pain. In complete tears, severe continuous pain over the shoulder area is inevitable, even at rest. In partial tears, pain may occur during shoulder movements. Lying sideways on the affected shoulder may also be painful.

Tenderness is the painful sensation that takes place when touching the affected area. In rotator cuff tears, tenderness may be perceptible over a particular shoulder region and the affected and adjacent muscles.

For example, a supraspinatus tear can cause pain and tenderness on palpation over the front area of the shoulder ball as well as the upper part of the shoulder blade.

b) Snapping/ popping sound

An audible or palpable snapping sound is heard or felt at the time of the injury, especially in a complete muscle tear.

c) Swelling

Swelling can be seen over the shoulder region in acute (recent) rotator cuff tears.

d) Redness & Bruising (Ecchymosis)

Severe bruising can be seen in complete tears, whereas less-to-no bruising is apparent in partial tears.

e) Change in the contour of the shoulder

In complete muscle tears, the muscle rolls up to one end of its attachments. So, a ball-like prominence is evident in complete muscle tears. Partial, chronic (long term) muscle tears show muscle wastage.

f) Reduction of the shoulder range of motion

Mainly the movements performed by the torn muscle are impaired. In addition, movements that stretch the affected muscle are also impaired. Therefore, any and all movements of the shoulder might be affected due to one muscle tear.

For example, in supraspinatus tears the main limited movement is shoulder abduction as it is the function of the muscle. In addition, the internal and external rotations of the shoulder are also impaired as the supraspinatus muscle stretches during these movements.

g) Reduction of the power of the movements

This can occur due to either pain or weakness.

Pain might limit certain movements, especially moving the arm behind the back, carrying something heavy, or performing overhead activities such as combing your hair, reaching something on a shelf etc.

Weakness might cause poor quality movements, such as reducing the amount of weight one can carry with the affected side.

3) Diagnosis of a Rotator Cuff Tear

a) Physical Diagnosis

The signs and symptoms mentioned above help in suspecting a rotator cuff tear. Movement restriction of the shoulder can be determined by measuring the Range of Motion (ROM) of the shoulder using a goniometer. The power of a muscle exerted during a movement can be identified by Manual Muscle Testing (MMT).

In addition, several physical tests can be performed in diagnosing tears of the rotator cuff muscles. Some of these tests are mentioned below:

Press-Belly Test (for tears in the Subscapularis muscle):

Place hands on your stomach. Make sure that the wrists are not bent either way and that the elbows are away from the chest, keeping the forearms parallel to the body. Press the stomach strongly with your hands while the forearms, hands and elbows set in one vertical plane.

If this position cannot be maintained as the arms and elbows draw backwards and the wrists bend to exert the pressure over the stomach, it is susceptible that the Subscapularis muscle has been injured/torn.

Jobe's Test (for tears in Supraspinatus muscle):

The therapist will abduct the arm into 90^0 and cross-flex/bring it forward a bit (parallel to the plane of the scapula). The extended thumb should be facing down. The therapist will put force on the forearm and ask you to raise the hand against that pressure.

Pain over the shoulder during this procedure often indicates a Supraspinatus tear. The strength of the muscle can also be determined by this test.

The Automatic Recall Test in Internal Rotation (for tears in Infraspinatus muscle):

The therapist will slightly abduct the arm into 20^0 with the shoulder externally rotated 5^0. You will be asked to hold the position.

Inability to hold this position and the forearm coming to its neutral/internally rotated position is a positive sign, which indicates a tear in the Infraspinatus muscle.

The Bulge Sign (for tears in Infraspinatus & Teres Minor muscles):

Place the hand on the mouth.

Positive test is announced if you raise your elbow higher than the hand level. It indicates that the Infraspinatus and

Teres minor, which are the external rotators of the shoulder, are torn out completely.

b) Medical Diagnosis

Diagnostic imaging tests assist in identifying rotator cuff tears. They are namely:

- X-rays of the shoulder

- Ultra-Sound Scanning (USS) of the shoulder

- Magnetic Resonance Imaging (MRI) of the shoulder

- Arthrography of the Shoulder (a type of X-ray taken after injecting a contrast dye into the joint)

4) Treatment Strategies – Partial Tears

a) Phase 1

Main Objective: Pain relief and Protection

Duration: First week after the injury

Tasks:

- Carry out "PRICER" protocol (refer Chapter 4)

- Discourage "HARM" protocol (refer Chapter 4)

- Medication for pain relief and inflammation reduction (Analgesics can be used for pain relief. NSAIDs help in reducing the inflammation. It is advisable to avoid anti-inflammatory medication during the first 2-3 days because they may promote further bleeding.)

- Postural and movement awareness to minimize further damage (Postural and movement limitations have to be acknowledged so as to prevent the pain from aggravating movements and postures.)

- Supportive slings to immobilize the injured shoulder (E.g.: Arm sling with shoulder abduction pillow)

b) Phase 2

Main Objective: Regain the shoulder mobility and prevent stiffness

Duration: 1 – 6 weeks after the injury

It will take at least 6 weeks to heal a rotator cuff tear. At the end of the healing process, muscle tissue is replaced with scar tissue. Scar tissue is not a stretchable structure. Therefore it can be subject to re-rupture.

Nevertheless, other shoulder muscles and the shoulder joint capsule may develop short-term or long-term protective tightness. This tightness also limits the movements of the shoulder.

Thus, it is essential to lengthen and smooth the healing scar tissue as well as the joint capsule and shoulder muscles. All of these activities should be in pain-free range.

Tasks:

- Perform massage (friction/kneading) to lengthen and smooth the healing scar tissue

- Carry out stretching exercises to lengthen the capsule and muscles of the back of the shoulder and the armpit

(One stretch should hold up to 1 minute. 10 such stretches should be carried out in one session. 3 sessions per day, every day)

Stretch Ext Exe 1 (Chapter 7)

Stretch Add/HAdd Exe 1 (Chapter 7)

Stretch Capsule Exe 1 (Chapter 7)

Stretch Capsule Exe 2 (Chapter 7)

- Perform active assisted movements of the shoulder to maintain muscle properties and prevent stiffness (Shoulder flexion, extension, abduction, medical rotation and lateral rotation)

c) Phase 3

Main Objective: Regain the scapular mobility

Duration: 1 – 6 weeks after the injury

This phase overlaps with Phase 2 and 4.

Scapula is responsible for two thirds of the movements of the shoulder. Normal shoulder blade-shoulder movement, medically termed as gleno-humeral rhythm, denotes proper gradient (2:1) of the scapula and humerus. It is essential for powerful shoulder function. Change of this movement pattern results in impingement and subsequent injury.

Tasks:

- Carry out scapular stabilization exercises to maintain scapular mobility

Scap Stabilize Exe 1 (Chapter 7)

Scap Stabilize Exe 2 (Chapter 7)

Scap Stabilize Exe 3 (Chapter 7)

Scap Stabilize Exe 4 (Chapter 7)

Scap Stabilize Exe 5 (Chapter 7)

Scap Stabilize Exe 6 (Chapter 7)

Scap Stabilize Exe 7 (Chapter 7)

- Reduce spasm and tightness of the Neck-Scapulo-Thoracic-Shoulder muscles (Through heat therapy and massage)

- Postural and movement awareness to minimize postural defects (Postural and movement limitations have to be acknowledged so as to prevent the shoulder from pain aggravating movements and postures.)

d) Phase 4

Main Objective: Regain normal Neck-Scapulo-Thoracic-Shoulder Function

Duration: 1 – 6 weeks after the injury

This phase overlaps with Phase 2 and 3.

The scapula and the thoracic cage form a false joint, though it contributes to the movements of the shoulder. This scapulo-thoracic joint is involved in moving the shoulder forwards and backwards. Most of the time, with injury of the shoulder joint, the scapulo-thoracic joint also gets stiffened. Normal gleno-humeral rhythm is disturbed in this case.

As the thoracic cage is attached to the spine, there might be stiffness in the neck and upper back vertebral joints as well.

Tasks:

- Undergo joint manipulative techniques to reduce/prevent stiffness (This needs hands-on-experience. A physiotherapist/chiropractic must be proficient in these tasks)

- Reduce spasm and tightness of the Neck-Scapulo-Thoracic-Shoulder muscles (Through heat therapy and massage)

- Perform prescribed exercises to maintain Neck-Scapulo-Thoracic-Shoulder function

- Postural and movement awareness to minimize postural defects (Postural and movement limitations have to be acknowledged as to prevent the shoulder from pain aggravating movements and postures.)

e) Phase 5

Main Objective: Increase rotator cuff strength

Duration: 3 – 8 weeks after the injury

According to the newest protocols, strengthening the rotator cuff muscles is not a task to be done at the final stage of rehabilitation.

Prior strengthening the muscles, it is compulsory to make sure that primary healing has taken place. Only then a muscle can be loaded and perform anti-gravity and resistance exercises.

Tasks:

- Perform adequate stretching exercises before doing strengthening exercises. (Refer Chapter 7)

- Carry out progressive strengthening exercises to regain the strength of rotator cuff muscles. (Refer Chapter 7)

f) Phase 6

Main Objective: Condition the rotator cuff muscles according to the work/sport performed

Duration: 3 – 8 weeks after the injury

Conditioning the partially torn rotator cuff muscle/s and the other compensatory muscles is essential to lead your normal active life. Strengthening is not sufficient for that.

For example, if you are a sportsman who performs javelin/putt you need to gain not only the power, but also the speed, agility and coordination to carry out the sport better.

Based on the requirements of the sport or occupation, particular sport-specific or work-specific exercises and a progressed training regime will be required to facilitate a safe and injury-free return to the chosen sport or employment. It is more advisable to have the guidance of a physiotherapist or a rehabilitation specialist, as he/she will specifically focus on your job or sport. He/She will discuss the goals, time scales and training schedules to optimize a complete return to the sport or work.

Tasks:

- Perform the sport-specific or work-specific exercise regime as prescribed by the physiotherapist/rehabilitation specialist. (Refer Chapter 6)

5) Treatment Strategies – Complete Tears

a) Phase 1

Main Objective: Pain relief and protection

Duration: First week after the injury

Carry out "PRICER" protocol and discourage "HARM" protocol (refer Chapter 4).

Medication can be used for pain relief and inflammation reduction. Mainly analgesics and NSAIDs can be helpful. It is advisable to avoid anti-inflammatory medication during the first 2-3 days because they may promote further bleeding.

Postural and movement limitations have to be acknowledged as to prevent the shoulder from pain aggravating movements and postures.

Supportive slings such as an arm sling with a shoulder abduction pillow are used to immobilize the injured shoulder.

b) Phase 2

Main Objective: Surgical Correction

Duration: 4 – 6 weeks after the injury

Complete muscle/tendon tear has no other option than surgery. Nevertheless, tears with unresolved symptoms that have not improved by exercises over 6-12 months, tears that are wider than 3 cm, and tears that cause prolonged weakness and/or loss of functions are also indicative of needed surgery.

There are 3 types of surgeries.

1. Arthroscopic surgery

The surgeon makes very small cuts of millimeters long in the shoulder and inserts a camera device called an "arthroscope". According to the view obtained from the arthroscope, the surgeon performs the necessary procedures with the aid of miniature surgical devices.

2. Open surgery

This is the traditional method of performing a surgery. An open surgical incision of several centimeters is made during the procedure. Deltoid muscle is often detached to see and obtain better access to the torn rotator cuff muscles/ tendons. The rehabilitation period in open surgeries is much longer than in arthroscopic procedures.

3. Mini-open surgery

Assessment of the degree of the injury is done via an arthroscpoe inserted into the muscles. After evaluating the damage, the repairing procedure is decided. The surgeon then makes an incision of 3 – 5 cm long to insert the surgical devices for the tendon/muscle repair. In this procedure, detachment of the deltoid is not necessary.

c) Phase 3 (Post surgical rehabilitation 1)

Main Objective: Maintain the shoulder mobility after immobilization

Duration: first 4 – 6 weeks after surgery

During the first few weeks, the main priority goes to protect the surgical site. Hence active movements have to be discouraged and the arm should be immobilized in a sling/cast. The period of immobilization is decided by the surgeon, depending on the surgical procedure performed.

When the surgeon gives permission to use the shoulder, passive exercises can be started. Passive exercises promote the shoulder mobility and maintain the range of motion of the shoulder. The physiotherapist will help in performing passive exercises. He/she will support the arm and move it in different directions that are safer and do not overstretch the surgical site. At the later stages of this phase, passive exercises can be progressed to active assisted exercises.

e) Phase 4 (Post surgical rehabilitation 2)

Main Objective: Regain the strength of the shoulder musculature

Duration: 6 weeks onwards after surgery

After 6 weeks, active exercises can be started. Active movements enhance the strength of the muscles as well as the coordination of the arm and the upper limb.

By the 8th week, a regime of strengthening exercises can be started. By this time, the repaired rotator cuff muscles may have healed adequately and may be ready to work as they did previously.

Complete recovery after a surgical repair of a rotator cuff tear may take several months. The normal duration of full recovery after a surgery is 4 – 6 months.

6) Home Management

In an acute injury;

- Use a bag of crushed ice or frozen peas to cool down the area for 20 minutes in 2 hourly intervals for the first 2-3 days. (Remember: Direct application of ice may induce frostbites. So the best practice is to place a thin towel over the treatment area while treating with ice.)

- Rest the shoulder in a sling, avoiding any movements of the shoulder that would increase the damage.

- Use a compressive garment to prevent swelling.

In a chronic tear;

- Use a hot pack or a hydro collator pack to heat up the area. InfraRed Therapy (if possible) can also be used for this purpose. Heat therapy needs to be applied for 20 minutes, 3 sessions per day on a daily basis. (Remember: It is necessary to keep a thin towel over the treatment area to prevent burns, especially when treating with hot packs or heating pads.)

- Do mobilization exercises to avoid stiffness of the shoulder. (Refer Chapter 7)

- Stretch the shoulder muscles appropriately. (Refer Chapter 7)

- Perform strengthening exercises in correct duration. (Refer Chapter 7)

- If there are no signs of healing, seek further medical interpretation.

7) Advice

- Once met with an injury, avoid moving the affected part.

- The best treatment in the first 3 days of an injury is ice.

- Don't rub or heat up the area within the first 3 days of the injury.

- Cover the area with a thin towel when you apply heat or ice.

- Avoid overhead activities and sudden jerky movements until the tear is healed properly.

- Avoid twisting movements of the shoulder.

After surgery;

- The elbow should bend at a 90^0 angle when resting in a sling.

- Always move the fingers, hand and wrist. At least 3 or 4 sessions of 10 – 15 repetitions should be done.

- Do not move your arm away from the body until the surgeon asks you to do so.

- Do not sleep lying flat. Keep a thin pillow to raise the shoulder.

- Do not lift anything with the repaired arm.

- Do not lean on the repaired arm.

- Do not move or twist the elbow backward to reach for things behind you.

Be alert for signs of medical emergency that needs special medical care:

- Excessive bleeding that does not stop when pressure is applied.

- Severe pain that does not respond to pain medications.

- Marked swelling of the arm.

- Numbness or burning/shock like sensation in the fingers and hands.

- Redness over the affected area.

- Pus (yellowish discharge) from the wounds.

- High fever (than 101^0 F).

- Dark discoloration of the hand, fingers, or fingernails.

- Coldness of the hand when compared to the non-affected hand.

8) Prognosis

Partial rotator cuff tears can be successfully treated through non-operative management, which includes painkillers, subacromial injections and physical therapy.

In very rare cases, especially in complete tears, surgery can be helpful.

The amount of time to recover differs from patient to patient according to their medical history. Partial tears that have a recent history would take less recovery time, most probably a couple of weeks. Complete tears that undergo surgery will have a 3 – 6 months rehabilitation period.

Chapter 9) Rotator Cuff Strain

Muscle fibers are stretchable and have the ability of contracting and relaxing. These fibers, in some circumstances, elongate more than they are supposed to. Damages occurred by overstretching the muscles are termed as muscle strains. Most of these overstretched muscles can be torn, as the external force applied is unbearable for the muscle.

Strains are of 3 stages:

Grade I Strain: Mild Muscle Strain

Less than 5% of the muscle fibres are damaged. Mild pain is experienced with no or minor swelling. Hence swelling is not a preliminary factor. There will not be any movement restriction due to pain.

The rest period needed for Grade I strain is 2 to 3 weeks.

Grade II Strain: Moderate Muscle Strain

Damage to the muscle fibres is worse, which results in partial muscle tear. More muscle fibres are involved than the Grade I strain, but the muscle is not completely ruptured. Moderate pain with swelling is evident. There is tenderness over the affected area. Bruising can be seen.

The rest period needed for Grade II strain is usually between 3 and 6 weeks.

Grade III Strain: Severe Muscle Strain

Complete rupture of a muscle falls under the category of Grade III strains. These strains/complete tears need surgical interventions to repair the muscle.

The rehabilitation period after a surgery is around 3 months.

All muscle strains should be rested and allowed to heal. If the patient continues to move, the condition will worsen. If ignored, a grade one strain has the potential to become a grade two strain or even a complete rupture.

Rotator cuff strains share the similar prevalence as rotator cuff tears. Rotator cuff strains also directly associate with age. There is no gender difference of acquisition in biological terms, although it is men who perform more hard work than women and therefore tears and strains are more apparent in men.

As a rotator cuff tear, which is the Grade III strain, has been discussed in the previous chapter; this chapter excludes complete tears (Grade III strains) to avoid duplication.

1) Causes & Risk Factors

Causes of rotator cuff strains are the same as the causes of tears. They include:

- A sudden thrust on the arm/shoulder

- A sudden force derived from the shoulder muscles

- Vigorous overhead activities

- Repetitive activities of the shoulder

- Certain sports such as baseball, tennis, badminton, squash, and cricket

- Normal wear and tear

Risk factors for a rotator cuff strain are as follows:

- Being more than 40 years old

- Lifting heavy objects

- Being a sportsman (especially baseball, tennis, and cricket players)

- Working in the construction field (especially carpenters, and painters)

- Poor postural adherence (especially rounded shoulders)

- Having weak shoulder muscles (could be due to inactivity or a previous trauma)

2) Signs & Symptoms

a) Pain and Tenderness

- Pain during shoulder movements

- Pain when lying down sideways on the affected shoulder

- Tenderness over the particular shoulder region and the affected and adjacent muscles

b) Muscle spasm

- Mainly in upper trapezius (shoulder blade muscle)

- Sometimes in paravertebral muscles (muscles beside the spine)

c) Swelling

Swelling over the shoulder region

d) Muscle wastage of the shoulder

Muscle wastage especially in partial, chronic muscle strains

e) Reduction of the shoulder range of motion

Shoulder flexion, extension, abduction, internal rotation and/or external rotation may get impaired depending on the strained muscle

f) Reduction of the power of the movements

- Moving the arm behind your back

- Carrying something heavy

- Performing overhead activities such as combing hair, reaching something on a shelf etc

3) Diagnosis of a Rotator Cuff Strain

a) Physical Diagnosis

Apart from the signs and symptoms mentioned above, several measurements and physical tests can be performed in diagnosing strains of the rotator cuff muscles.

Range of Motion (ROM) of the shoulder:

ROM can be measured using a goniometer. All the movements should be measured to identify impaired movements in low-grade strains.

Manual Muscle Testing (MMT) of the shoulder:

The power of each rotator cuff muscle can be tested and graded according to this system.

Press-Belly Test (for Subscapularis muscle):

Refer to test procedure and test interpretation in Chapter 8.

Jobe's Test (for Supraspinatus muscle):

Refer to test procedure and test interpretation in Chapter 8.

The Automatic Recall Test in Internal Rotation (for Infraspinatus muscle):

Refer to test procedure and test interpretation in Chapter 8.

The Bulge Sign (for Infraspinatus & Teres Minor muscles):

Refer to test procedure and test interpretation in Chapter 8.

b) Medical Diagnosis

The following diagnostic imaging tests assist in identifying rotator cuff strains:

- X-rays of the shoulder

- Ultra-Sound Scanning (USS) of the shoulder

- Magnetic Resonance Imaging (MRI) of the shoulder

- Arthrography of the Shoulder (a type of X-ray taken after injecting a contrast dye into the joint)

4) Treatment Strategies

a) Phase 1

Main Objective: Pain relief and Protection

Duration: First week after the injury

Tasks:

- Carry out "PRICER" protocol (refer Chapter 4)

- Discourage "HARM" protocol (refer Chapter 4)

- Analgesics and NSAIDs help in reducing pain and inflammation

- Postural and movement awareness to minimize further damage

- Supportive slings to immobilize the injured shoulder

b) Phase 2

Main Objective: Regain the shoulder mobility and prevent stiffness

Duration: 1 – 6 weeks after the injury

Tasks:

- Perform massage (friction/kneading) to lengthen and smooth the healing scar tissue

- Carry out stretching exercises to lengthen the capsule and muscles of the back of the shoulder and the armpit

Stretch Ext Exe 1 (Chapter 7)

Stretch Add/HAdd Exe 1 (Chapter 7)

Stretch Capsule Exe 1 (Chapter 7)

Stretch Capsule Exe 2 (Chapter 7)

- Perform active assisted movements of the shoulder (Shoulder flexion, extension, abduction, medical rotation and lateral rotation) to maintain muscle properties and prevent stiffness.

c) Phase 3

Main Objective: Regain the scapular mobility

Duration: 1 – 6 weeks after the injury

Tasks:

- Carry out scapular stabilization exercises to maintain scapular mobility

Scap Stabilize Exe 1 (Chapter 7)

Scap Stabilize Exe 2 (Chapter 7)

Scap Stabilize Exe 3 (Chapter 7)

Scap Stabilize Exe 4 (Chapter 7)

Scap Stabilize Exe 5 (Chapter 7)

Scap Stabilize Exe 6 (Chapter 7)

Scap Stabilize Exe 7 (Chapter 7)

- Reduce spasm and tightness of the Neck-Scapulo-Thoracic-Shoulder muscles

- Postural and movement awareness to minimize postural defects

d) Phase 4

Main Objective: Regain normal Neck-Scapulo-Thoracic-Shoulder Function

Duration: 1 – 6 weeks after the injury

Tasks:

- Undergo joint manipulative techniques to reduce/prevent stiffness carried out by a qualified professional

- Reduce spasm and tightness of the Neck-Scapulo-Thoracic-Shoulder muscles

- Perform prescribed exercises to maintain Neck-Scapulo-Thoracic-Shoulder function

- Postural and movement awareness to minimize postural defects

e) Phase 5

Main Objective: Increase rotator cuff strength

Duration: 3 – 8 weeks after the injury

Tasks:

- Perform adequate stretching exercises before doing strengthening exercises. (Refer to Chapter 7)

- Carry out progressive strengthening exercises to regain the strength of the rotator cuff muscles. (Refer to Chapter 7)

f) Phase 6

Main Objective: Condition the rotator cuff muscles according to the work/sport performed

Duration: 3 – 8 weeks after the injury

Tasks:

- Perform the sport-specific or work-specific exercise regime as prescribed by the physiotherapist/rehabilitation specialist. (Refer Chapter 7)

5) Home Management

In an acute strain;

- Use a bag of crushed ice or frozen peas to cool down the area for 20 minutes in 2 hourly intervals for the first 2-3 days. (Remember: Direct application of ice may induce frostbites. So the best practice is to place a thin towel over the treatment area while treating with ice.)

- Rest the shoulder in a sling, avoiding any movements of the shoulder that would increase the damage.

- Use a compressive garment to prevent swelling.

In a chronic strain;

- Use a hot pack or a hydro collator pack to heat up the area. InfraRed Therapy (if possible) can also be used in this purpose. Heat therapy needs to be carried out for 20 minutes, 3 sessions per day on daily basis.(Remember: It is necessary to keep a thin towel over the treatment area to prevent burns, especially when treating with hot packs or heating pads.)

- Do mobilization exercises to avoid stiffness of the shoulder. (Refer to Chapter 7)

- Stretch the shoulder muscles appropriately. (Refer to Chapter 7)

- Perform strengthening exercises in correct duration. (Refer to Chapter 7)

- If there are no signs of healing, seek for further medical interpretation.

6) Advice

- Once met with an injury, avoid moving the affected part.

- The best treatment in the first 3 days of an injury is ice.

- Don't rub or heat up the area within first 3 days of the injury.

- Cover the area with a thin towel when you apply heat or ice.

- Avoid overhead activities and sudden jerky movements.

- Avoid twisting movements of the shoulder.

Be alert for signs of a <u>medical emergency</u> that needs special medical care:

- Excessive bleeding that does not stop when pressure is applied.

- Severe pain that does not respond to pain medications.

- Marked swelling of the arm.

- Numbness or burning/shock like sensation in the fingers and hands.

- Redness over the affected area.

- High fever (than 101^0 F).

- Dark discoloration of the hand, fingers, or fingernails.

- Coldness of the hand when compared to the non-affected hand.

7) Prognosis

A combination of medication and physical therapy promotes full recovery after a rotator cuff strain. Very rarely, local intramuscular injections will be needed to reduce pain and therefore gain movements.

Chapter 10) Rotator Cuff Tendinopathy

Tendinopathy is an injury to the tendons. Rotator cuff muscles contribute four tendons to the shoulder joint. There can be an injury to any of these tendons.

Injuries to the tendons are of two types; tendinosis and tendonitis.

Tendinosis is having minor tears in the tendon. There can be some signs of inflammation, but they are not significant. This is the most common type of tendinopathy.

Tendonitis, also called as tendinitis, is the inflammatory condition of tendons. This is less common when compared to tendinosis, but as the cardinal signs of inflammation are significantly visible in tendinitis, it is in tendinitis that people are seeking medical advice, not in tendinosis.

All the tendons have the risk of getting injured and inflamed, but Supraspinatus tendinitis is the most common type of rotator cuff tendinopathy.

There is evidence saying that 1 in 50 adults have tendinopathy in the US. 0.95% of the UK population is suffering from shoulder pain where 85% of them were due to rotator cuff tears or tendinopathies . This prevalence increases with age.

Tendinopathies may progress into rotator cuff tears or calcified tendons in later stages if not properly treated.

1) Causes & Risk Factors

Main causes of tendinopathy include,

- Repetitive overhead activities
- Activities generating sudden force by shoulder musculature such as throwing
- Inflammatory conditions of the shoulder (e.g.: arthritis)
- Trauma to the shoulder
- Fall on outstretched hand
- Degenerative changes of the shoulder due to aging

Risk factors for developing tendinopathy comprise of:

- Being older than 30
- Playing racquet sports (e.g.: tennis, badminton)
- Performing overhead reaching occupations (e.g.: painting)

2) Signs & Symptoms

a) Pain and Tenderness

- Less degree of pain during movements and at rest in the initial stages
- Progress into 'toothache' like pain when performing reaching activities and/or lifting
- Pain radiating from the front of the shoulder to the

side of the mid-arm

- Pain aggravated when sleeping on the affected shoulder
- Pain increases in certain activities such as overhead reaching activities and reaching behind you
- Tenderness may be felt at the front and sides of the shoulder ball

b) Clicking sound

An audible or palpable 'click' when performing overhead activities

c) Swelling

Slight localized swelling over the shoulder.

d) Restriction of certain movements of the shoulder

- Reduction of the range of motion of the shoulder
- May be due to either pain or stiffness
- Difficulties in performing overhead activities
- Difficulties in reaching behind as to do up the buttons or the zip or fasten underclothing

e) Reduction of the power of the movements

- Can occur due to weakness
- Cause poor quality movements

3) Diagnosis of a Rotator Cuff Tendinopathy

a) Physical Diagnosis

Range of Motion (ROM) of the shoulder:

ROM can be measured using a goniometer. Recording this helps in assessing the progress of the treatment.

Manual Muscle Testing (MMT) of the shoulder:

The power of each rotator cuff muscle can be tested and graded in order to find weak muscles.

Press-Belly Test (for Subscapularis muscle):

Refer to test procedure and test interpretation in Chapter 8.

Jobe's Test (for Supraspinatus muscle):

Refer to test procedure and test interpretation in Chapter 8.

The Automatic Recall Test in Internal Rotation (for Infraspinatus muscle):

Refer to test procedure and test interpretation in Chapter 8.

The Bulge Sign (for Infraspinatus & Teres Minor muscles):

Refer to test procedure and test interpretation in Chapter 8.

b) Medical Diagnosis

Diagnostic imaging tests assist in identifying rotator cuff tears. They are namely:

- X-rays of the shoulder

- Ultra-Sound Scanning (USS) of the shoulder

- Magnetic Resonance Imaging (MRI) of the shoulder

- Arthrography of the Shoulder (a type of X-ray taken after injecting a contrast dye into the joint)

4) Treatment Strategies

a) Phase 1

Main Objective: Pain relief and Protection

Duration: First week after the injury

Tasks:

- Rest the affected shoulder in a sling. Avoid activities that worsen the shoulder pain.

- Cool the area by applying ice during the first 2-3 days or after exercises.

- Use heat after 3 days to reduce pain.

- Use analgesics and NSAIDs for pain relief and inflammation reduction.

- Postural and movement awareness to minimize further damage.

b) Phase 2

Main Objective: Regain the shoulder mobility and prevent stiffness

Duration: 1 – 6 weeks after the injury

Tasks:

- Perform friction to break down the adhesions and smooth the healing scar tissue within the tendon.

- Carry out stretching exercises to lengthen the capsule and muscles of the back of the shoulder and the armpit.

Stretch Ext Exe 1 (Chapter 7)

Stretch Add/HAdd Exe 1 (Chapter 7)

Stretch Capsule Exe 1 (Chapter 7)

Stretch Capsule Exe 2 (Chapter 7)

- Perform active assisted movements (Shoulder flexion, extension, abduction, medical rotation and lateral rotation) of the shoulder to maintain muscle properties and prevent stiffness.

c) Phase 3

Main Objective: Regain the scapular mobility

Duration: 1 – 6 weeks after the injury

Tasks:

- Carry out scapular stabilization exercises to maintain scapular mobility.

Scap Stabilize Exe 1 (Chapter 7)

Scap Stabilize Exe 2 (Chapter 7)

Scap Stabilize Exe 3 (Chapter 7)

Scap Stabilize Exe 4 (Chapter 7)

Scap Stabilize Exe 5 (Chapter 7)

Scap Stabilize Exe 6 (Chapter 7)

Scap Stabilize Exe 7 (Chapter 7)

- Reduce spasm and tightness of the Neck-Scapulo-Thoracic-Shoulder muscles.

- Postural and movement awareness to minimize postural defects.

d) Phase 4

Main Objective: Regain normal Neck-Scapulo-Thoracic-Shoulder Function

Duration: 1 – 6 weeks after the injury

Tasks:

- Undergo joint manipulative techniques performed by a qualified professional to reduce/prevent stiffness.

- Reduce spasm and tightness of the Neck-Scapulo-Thoracic-Shoulder muscles.

- Perform prescribed exercises to maintain Neck-Scapulo-Thoracic-Shoulder function.

- Postural and movement awareness to minimize postural defects.

e) Phase 5

Main Objective: Increase rotator cuff strength

Duration: 3 – 8 weeks after the injury

Tasks:

- Perform adequate stretching exercises before doing strengthening exercises. (Refer Chapter 7)

- Carry out progressive strengthening exercises to regain the strength of rotator cuff muscles. (Refer Chapter 7)

f) Phase 6

Main Objective: Condition the rotator cuff muscles according to the work/sport performed

Duration: 3 – 8 weeks after the injury

Tasks:

- Perform the sport-specific or work-specific exercise regime as prescribed by the physiotherapist/rehabilitation specialist. (Refer to Chapter 7)

Surgical interventions are performed in severe injuries. It involves repairing the tendon by suturing it to the bone (e.g.: humerus).

5) Home Management

In an acute injury;

- Use a bag of crushed ice or frozen peas to cool down the area for 20 minutes in 2 hourly intervals for the first 2-3 days. (Remember: Direct application of ice may induce frostbites. So the best practice is to place a thin towel over the treatment area while treating with ice.)

- Rest the shoulder in a sling, avoiding any movements of the shoulder that would increase the damage.

In a chronic injury;

- Use a hot pack or a hydro collator pack to heat up the area. InfraRed Therapy (if possible) can also be used in this purpose. Heat therapy needs to be carried out for 20 minutes, 3 sessions per day on daily basis. (Remember: It is necessary to keep a thin towel over the treatment area to prevent burns, especially when treating with hot packs or heating pads.)

- Do mobilization exercises to avoid stiffness of the shoulder. (Refer to Chapter 7)

- Stretch the shoulder muscles appropriately. (Refer to Chapter 7)

- Perform strengthening exercises in correct duration. (Refer to Chapter 7)

- If there are no signs of healing, seek for further medical interpretation.

6) Advice

- Once met with an injury, avoid moving the affected part.

- The best treatment in the first 3 days of an injury is ice.

- Don't rub or heat up the area within first 3 days of the injury.

- Cover the area with a thin towel when you apply heat or ice.

- Avoid overhead activities and sudden jerky movements.

- Avoid twisting movements of the shoulder.

- Change job duties if you are to perform overhead activities.

- Never ever try to work ignoring the shoulder pain.

- Do not increase exercise duration or intensity more than 10% per week.

Be alert for signs of a medical emergency that needs special medical care:

- Severe pain that does not respond to pain medications.

- Marked swelling of the arm.

- Numbness or burning/shock like sensation in the fingers and hands.

- Redness over the affected area.

- High fever (than 101^0 F).

- Dark discoloration of the hand, fingers, or fingernails.

- Coldness of the hand when compared to the non-affected hand.

7) Prognosis

Rotator cuff tendinitis is often associated with shoulder bursitis and bicipital tendinitis. It may progress into calcified tendons or rotator cuff tears if not treated properly.

Physiotherapy together with pain medication promotes better prognosis.

Chapter 11) Rotator Cuff Bursitis

Bursa is a fluid filled bag demarcated by a synovial membrane. It cushions the space between bones and tendons and/or muscles. There are 3 main bursae in the shoulder joint. Subacromial/subdeltoid bursa is the main bursa in shoulder. It is located in between the deltoid muscle and the coraco-acromial arch, reducing the friction during the forceful movements.

Bursitis is an inflammation of the bursae. If not properly treated, it might end up being a calcified bursa.

It has a gradual onset.

1) Causes & Risk Factors

Main causes of rotator cuff bursitis include:

- Overuse of the shoulder joint

- Direct trauma to the shoulder

- Fall on outstretched hand

- Inflammatory conditions of the shoulder (e.g.: arthritis)

In some cases, there is no particular cause evident for the occurrence of bursitis. Such cases are called idiopathic.

2) Signs & Symptoms

Pain and Tenderness

- Pain on the outer side of the shoulder

- Pain radiating from the shoulder to the elbow or wrist

- Pain is aggravated when sleeping on the affected shoulder

- Pain increases when the arm is abducted in between 60^0 and 120^0 ("Painful arc")

- Pain reduces at the final degrees of abduction

- Pain aggravates in overhead reaching activities such as combing hair and reaching a higher shelf of the cupboard

- Tenderness over the outer side of the shoulder

Swelling

Localized swelling over the shoulder if severely inflamed

Redness

Redness over the outer side of the shoulder joint if severely inflamed

Restriction of certain movements of the shoulder

- Limitation of shoulder abduction

- Difficulties in performing overhead activities

Reduction of the power of the movements

Cause poor quality movements, especially abduction

3) Diagnosis of a Rotator Cuff Bursitis

a) Physical Diagnosis

Range of Motion (ROM) of the shoulder:

ROM of shoulder abduction, flexion, extension, internal rotation and external rotation has to be measured.

Manual Muscle Testing (MMT) of the shoulder:

The power of each rotator cuff muscle can be tested and graded in order to find weak muscles.

Neer's Sign:

You will be asked to do forward elevation of the internally rotated arm above 90°.

If pain is present, it is considered a positive sign. This will identify impingement of the rotator cuff but is also sensitive for subacromial bursitis.

Resisted adduction:

The therapist will fully abduct your shoulder. Then the therapist will ask you to lower the arm while he/she resists the movement.

Persistence of the pain during the resisted adduction indicates subacromial bursitis. Pain diminishes if you are having supraspinatus tendinitis.

b) Medical Diagnosis

Diagnostic imaging tests that assist in identifying bursitis are:

- X-rays of the shoulder

- Ultra-Sound Scanning (USS) of the shoulder

- Magnetic Resonance Imaging (MRI) of the shoulder

- Arthrography of the Shoulder (a type of X-ray taken after injecting a contrast dye into the joint)

4) Treatment Strategies

There are 2 types of treatment strategies: conservative and surgical management.

a) Conservative Management

- "PRICE" Protocol

- Pain medication (e.g.: NSAIDs, Analgesics)

- Corticosteroid injections (e.g.: hydrocortisone, dexamethasone, prednisolone)

- Antibiotics to control inflammation

- Codman's mobilization exercises to prevent stiffness of the shoulder (Refer to Chapter 7)

- Scapular exercises to maintain mobility of the scapula (Refer to Scap Stabilize Exe 1-2 in Chapter 7)

- Perform stretching exercises to the tight muscles. (Refer to Chapter 7)

- Strengthening exercises to regain the strength of rotator cuff muscles. (Refer to Chapter 7)

b) Surgical Management

- Very rare

- Performed as drainage through incision, excision of the bursa with chronic inflammation and removal of problematic bony prominences

- Pain medication (eg: NSAIDs, Analgesics) are used at the initial days after surgery

- Rehabilitation program is carried out as the rotator cuff tear repairs (Refer to Chapter 8)

5) Home Management

In an acute injury;

- Use a bag of crushed ice or frozen peas to cool down the area for 20 minutes in 2 hourly intervals for the first 2-3 days.

- Rest the shoulder in a sling, avoiding any movements of the shoulder that would increase the damage.

In a chronic injury;

- Use a hot pack or a hydro collator pack to heat up the area. InfraRed Therapy (if possible) also can be used in this purpose. Heat therapy needs to be carried out for 20 minutes, 3 sessions per day on daily basis.

- Visit the doctor if the pain is severe, to obtain subacromial injections of local anaesthetics and corticosteroids.

- Do mobilization exercises to avoid stiffness of the shoulder. (Refer to Chapter 6)

- Stretch the shoulder muscles appropriately. (Refer to Chapter 6)

- Perform strengthening exercises in correct duration. (Refer to Chapter 6)

- If there are no signs of healing, seek for further medical interpretation.

6) Advice

- Avoid overhead activities and sudden jerky movements.

- Avoid twisting movements of the shoulder.

- Change job duties if you are to perform overhead activities.

- Never ever try to work ignoring the shoulder pain.

- Do not increase exercise duration or intensity more than 10% per week.

Be alert for signs of a medical emergency that needs special medical care:

- Severe pain that does not respond to pain medications.

- Marked swelling of the arm.

- Numbness or burning/ shock like sensation in the fingers and hands.

- Redness over the affected area.

- High fever (than 101^0 F).

- Dark discoloration of the hand, fingers, or fingernails.

- Coldness of the hand when compared to the non-affected hand.

7) Prognosis

Rotator cuff bursitis is associated with rotator cuff tendinitis and bicipital tendinitis. It may progress into calcified bursa if not treated properly.

Physiotherapy treatments help in relieving the pain and reducing the joint stiffness. The inflammation of the bursa has to subside immediately with medication and local injections.

Chapter 12) Alternative Therapies

In an attempt to find relief from their symptoms, many people will start to look to alternative therapies. While many of these treatments can be beneficial in many ways, most of these treatments are designed to be complimentary and aren't meant to take the place of traditional medicine.

If you wish to try some of the alternative therapies available, then consult a doctor first. Moreover, when looking for alternative treatments, do your research carefully and follow these tips when looking for a practitioner: Be aware that some therapies might make your condition worse if given the wrong advice/treatment.

Make sure that the person you are planning to see is fully qualified to treat you and your condition. Moreover, do some careful research first to find out the success rates of your treatment of choice.

If doing any of the alternative therapies described below gives you a lot of pain, stop immediately and consult your doctor before continuing.

1) Acupuncture

Acupuncture works by placing needles into the skin to release blocked energy or chi. It is thought that acupuncture works by triggering the release of pain-reducing opioids. It shouldn't be used by patients on blood thinning medications or by patients with a blood clotting disorder.

The word "Acupuncture" means "prick with a needle". It is an ancient Chinese therapeutic intervention. It involves inserting needles in to very specific points of the skin called acupoints. It is an effective non-pharmacological treatment technique for many diseases.

According to Chinese medicine, Qi – The Vital Energy of the body, flows in the pathways located along "meridians". These energy channels are believed to be connected to the internal organs of the body. Needles are used either to increase or decrease the flow of energy, or to unblock the flow of energy if it has been obstructed.

2) Tai Chi

If you are usually an active person, it can be frustrating to wait until you are able to return to your usual sports and activities. However, while you are waiting to get back into the sports you enjoy, there is an ideal opportunity to try something new.

Tai Chi is a slow paced form of exercise, but it can be every bit as challenging. Tai Chi is often described as meditation in motion, and the slow, smooth moves of Tai Chi certainly have a calming influence on the mind.

Tai Chi can also help to improve mobility, co-ordination and balance.

Chi Kung and Qi Qing also offers a gentle form of exercise to keep the mind and body active, and provide a good way of exercising while waiting to get back into normal exercise. The graceful movements of these types of meditative movements are a good alternative to stronger paced exercises and it would be a good idea to practice these forms of exercise more often once you do get back to your usual exercise routine in order to provide a contrast to your usual workouts and give the tendons and muscles a much needed rest as well as giving them an additional challenge.

3) Osteopathy

By using manipulation techniques, osteopaths believe that this technique can enable the body to heal itself. Osteopathy is often used for the treatment of sports injuries.

4) Alexander Technique

The Alexander Technique teaches patients how to reduce tension in their bodies. The technique helps people to walk better, stand better and to use their bodies in a safer, healthier way to avoid strain or stress.

People who use the Alexander Technique often say that, after years of pain and discomfort, they are able to walk freely and comfortably after practicing the technique.

5) Pilates

Pilates is essentially a mind-body technique. It involves very slow, small movements that encourage you to think about each muscle as you use it.

6) Chiropractic Therapy

A chiropractor is trained to help treat with the neuro musculoskeletal system. The emphasis is on releasing the joints, however, some patients with rotator cuff problems might find this type of treatment useful for their condition, as it will act to release tension throughout the body.

7) Trigger Point Therapy

Trigger Point Therapy is often used by therapists to reduce pain. The technique can be used to relieve all sorts of painful conditions including the pain caused by overuse injuries.

While many people find this an effective way of managing their pain, it should also be noted that with some people pressing on trigger points can make the pain worse. Unfortunately, the only way to determine if you will be one of the patients from this sore of treatment is by trying it.

Some people will experience a momentary soreness before finding relief, while others find that the pain takes longer to go away, but that this technique does work for them.

If this kind of treatment interests you, you'll find many books available on the subject.

Chapter 13) Devices Used In Rotator Cuff Injuries

1) Devices Used for Pain Relief

a) Cold Compression Wrap

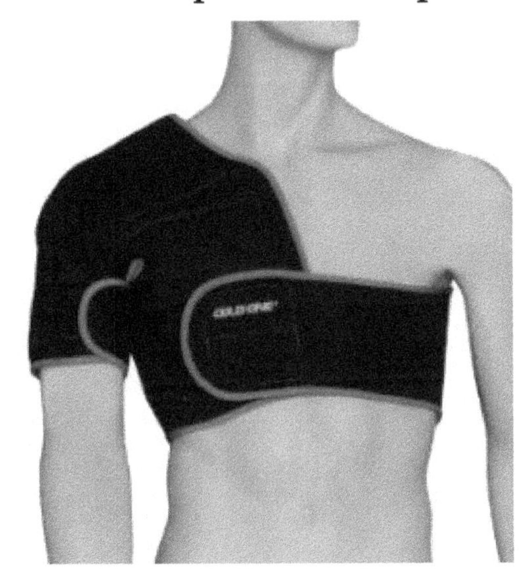

Source: www.amazon.com

Features:

- It reduces inflammation and pain by cryotherapy (cold therapy).

- It helps to reduce swelling by compression.

Indications:

Acute rotator cuff injury

Where to Buy:

Cold One® Shoulder Ice Compression Wrap –

Cold One Official Store www.coldone.com

Amazon www.amazon.com

King Brand® ColdCure® Wrap –

King Brand Healthcare Products Ltd
(http://kingbrand.com/Shoulder-Wraps.php)

Talar Made Cold Compress Shoulder Wrap –

FIRSTAID4SPORT www.firstaid4sport.co.uk

2) Devices Used in Immobilization

a) Shoulder Sling

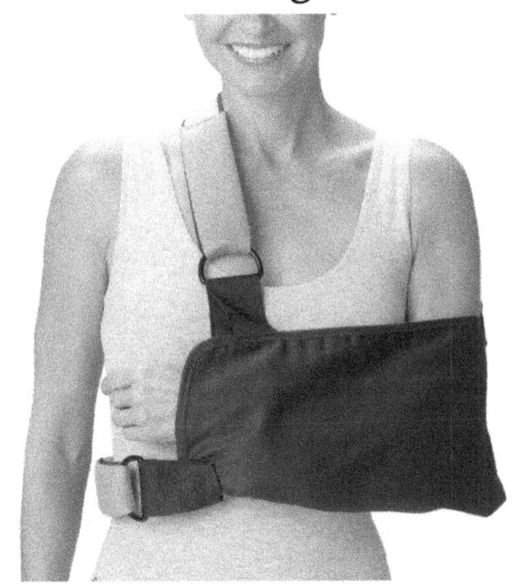

Source: www.Amazon.co.uk

Features:

- It immobilizes the shoulder to allow healing following shoulder injuries.

- It helps in stabilizing the shoulder following shoulder surgeries where shoulder movements are prohibited.

Indications:

Rotator cuff repair

Where to Buy:

ProCare Shoulder Sling (with foam straps)

ebay www.ebay.co.uk

Amazon www.amazon.co.uk

PhysioRoom www.physioroom.com

Thermoskin Arm Sling

Health and Care www.healthandcare.co.uk

b) Sling and Swathe

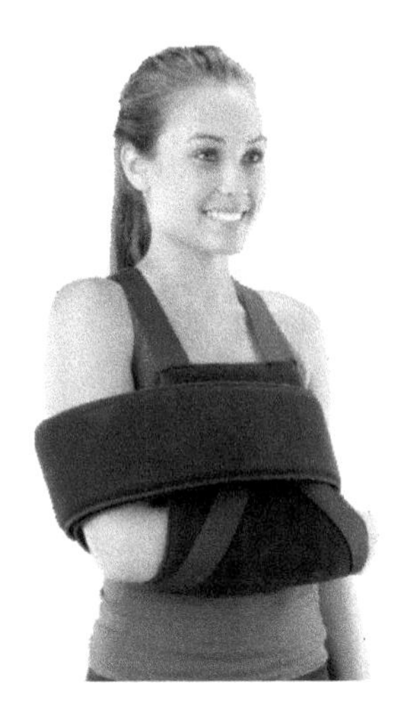

Source: www.Amazon.com

Features:

- Light weighted support.

- It immobilizes the upper extremity after trauma.

- Complete shoulder immobilization can be achieved.

Indications:

- Neurological conditions such as paralysis or hemiplegia

- Rotator Cuff Repair or Capsular Shift

- Glenohumeral Dislocation or Subluxation

- Bankhart Repair (to prevent anterior dislocation of the shoulder)

- Soft Tissue Strains or Repairs

Where to Buy:

Sling and Swathe Universal –

Breg www.breg.com

Amazon www.amazon.com

Bledsoe Sling and Swathe Immobilizer –

Bledsoe www.bledsoebrace.com

c) Arm Sling with Shoulder Abduction Pillow

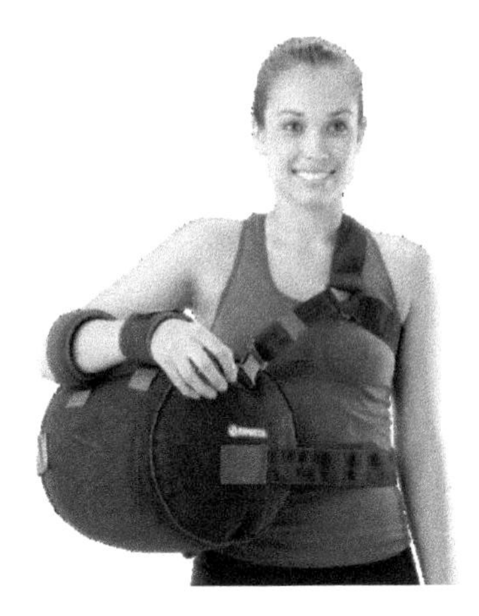

Source: www.Amazon.co.uk

Features:

It consists of a contoured pillow that maintains the shoulder in abduction. The degree of abduction is adjustable.

Indications:

- SLAP lesion repairs
- Bankart repairs
- Rotator cuff repairs
- Shoulder separations
- Shoulder dislocations

Where to Buy:

Shoulder Abduction Pillow –

Breg www.breg.com

Amazon www.amazon.com

Bledsoe Original ARC with Pillow –

Bledsoe www.bledsoebrace.com

d) Shoulder Support Strap

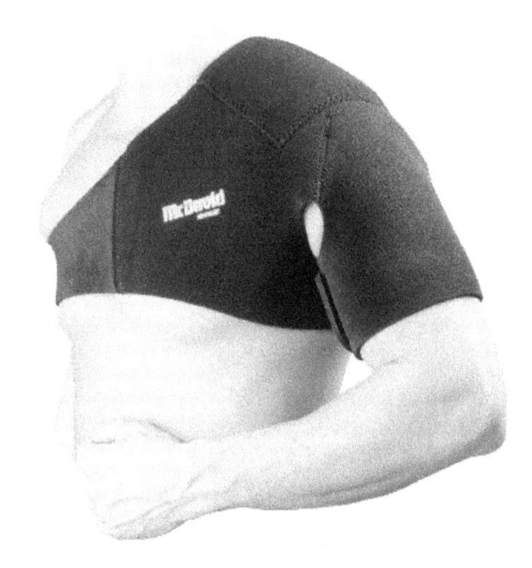

Source: www.Amazon.com

Features:

It reduces shoulder pain and stiffness by retaining heat.

Indications:

- Shoulder bursitis
- Rotator cuff injury
- Impingement syndrome
- Tendonitis
- Myositis

Where to Buy:

McDavid Universal Shoulder Support –

PhysioRoom www.physioroom.com

Amazon www.amazon.com

PhysioRoom Shoulder Support Neoprene Therapy Strap/Brace –

Ebay www.ebay.co.uk

e) Mueller Shoulder Brace

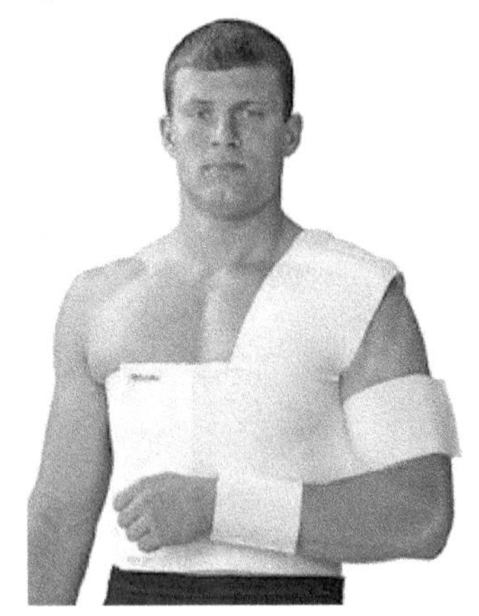

Source: www.Amazon.co.uk

Features:

- It immobilizes the shoulder and arm to promote healing in shoulder separation.

- It provides support for the shoulder joint.

- It helps to prevent re-injury when returning to sport activities after the ligament has healed.

Indications:

Acromio-Clavicular joint sprain (shoulder separation)

Where to Buy:

Mueller Sports Medicine www.muellersportsmed.com

Amazon www.amazon.com

PhysioRoom www.physioroom.com

f) OmoTrain Shoulder Support

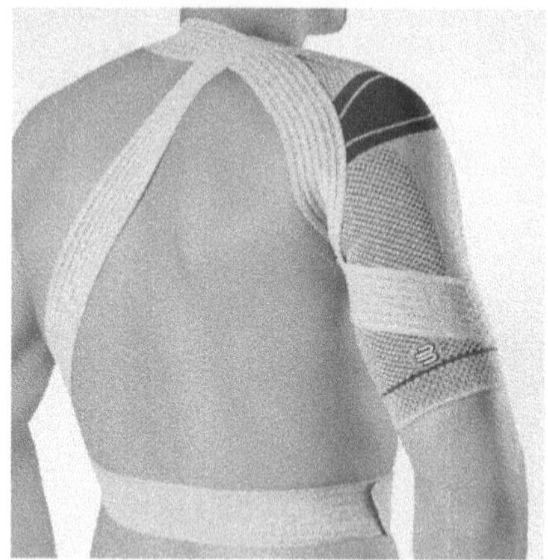

Source: www.Amazon.com

Features:

- It relieves shoulder pain.

- It stabilizes the shoulder and provides guidance through movements performed.

- It gives re-assurance following injuries to the shoulder.

Indications:

- Frozen shoulder

- Osteoarthritis

- Dislocated shoulder

- Broken collarbone

- Rotator Cuff injuries and repairs

- Acromio-Clavicular injuries

Where to Buy:

Bauerfeind OmoTrain Shoulder Support –

Bauerfeind www.bauerfeind.com

PhysioRoom www.physioroom.com

Amazon www.amazon.com

g) Sully Shoulder Stabilizer

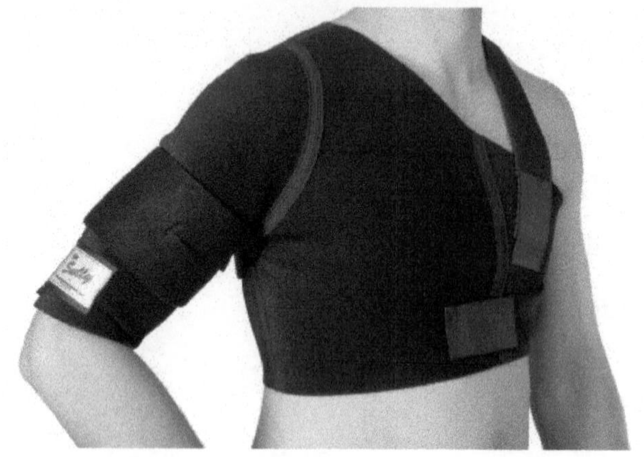

Source: www.Amazon.com

Features:

- It pulls the humerus backward while it restricts external rotation and abduction.

- Its elastic straps attach with Velcro at any point, in any direction and with any amount of force.

- The smooth, controlled assistance or restraint follows the natural movement of the muscles and joints.

Indications:

- Rotator Cuff repairs

- Glenohumeral dislocations

- Soft tissue strains and repairs

- Acromio-Clavicular injuries

Where to Buy:

DJO Global www.djoglobal.com

Donjoy International www.donjoy.eu

Amazon www.amazon.com

3) Assistive Devices Used in Facilitating Movements

a) Reachers

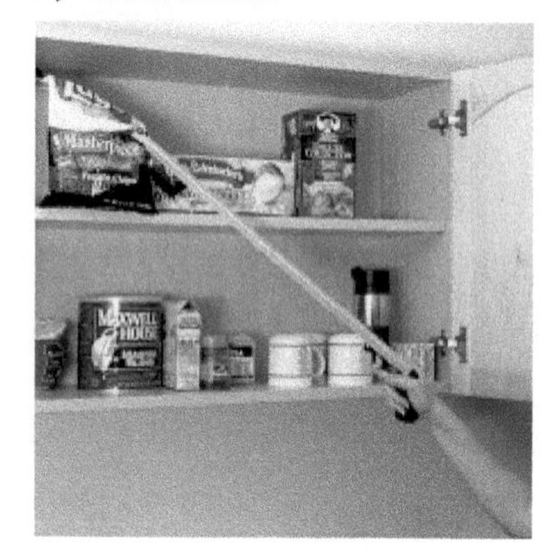

Source: www.walgreens.com

Features:

Reachers are ideal for people with a limited range of motion or difficulty bending

Perfect for picking up objects as small as a dime and as large as a quart bottle

Slip-resistant, ergonomic, contoured handle

Indications:

- Rotator cuff injuries

- Back and neck injuries

Where to Buy:

Essential Medical Standard Reacher –

Walgreens www.walgreens.com

Mabis Aluminum Reacher with Magnetic Tip 26 inch 26-inch –

Walgreens www.walgreens.com

b) Zipper Pulls

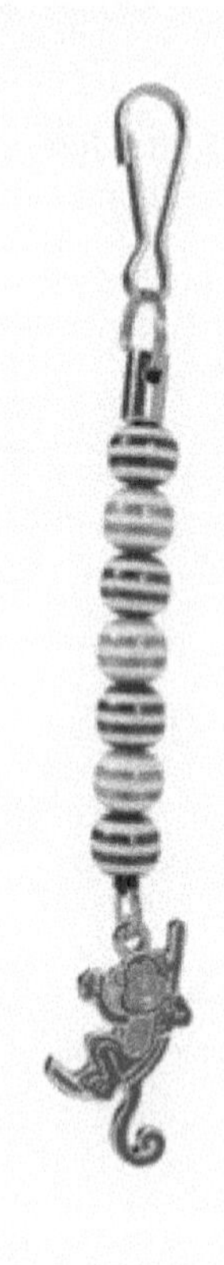

Source: www.Amazon.co.uk

Features:

Assistive device for people with shoulder pain

Perfect to be used on backpacks, jackets, lunchboxes, sweaters, suitcases, sport duffels, etc

Indications:

- Rotator cuff injuries

- Back and neck injuries

Where to Buy:

CoolZips www.coolzips.com

Amazon www.amazon.com

c) Curved Bath Brush

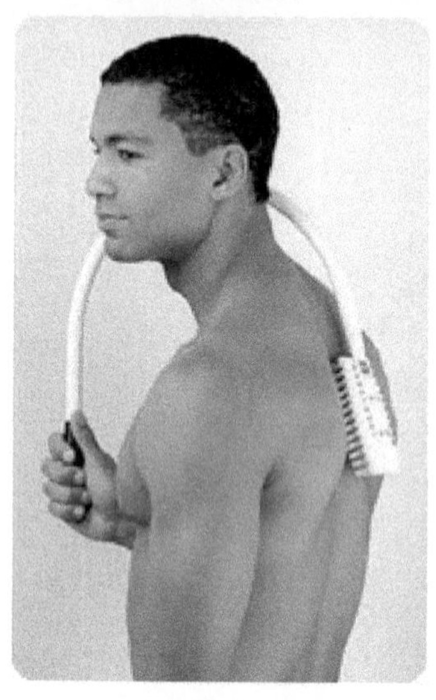

Source: www.techforltc.org

Features:

The Bendable Shower Brush is designed to enable those with limited range of motion to wash their back. Handle is curved 180^{0}.

Indications:

- Rotator cuff injuries

Where to Buy:

Technology for Long-Term-Care www.techforltc.org

d) Ableware® Roll Easy Lotion Applicator

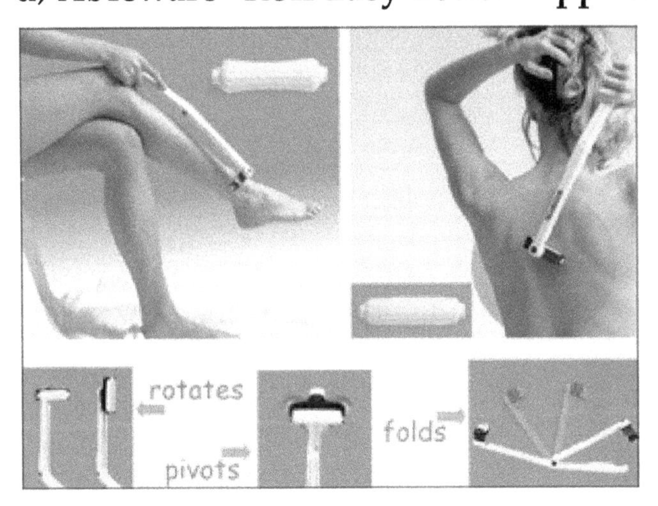

Source: www.techforltc.org

Features:

The Ableware® Roll Easy Lotion Applicator is designed to assist with applying moisturizing lotions, suntan oils, sport creams and medications on hard-to-reach places and massage the body while doing so. This device offers a pivoting head and comes with two different massage rollers. The inverted roller is for the arms, legs, and neck and the round roller is for use on the back. The handle folds for storage.

Indications:

- Rotator cuff injuries

Where to Buy:

Technology for Long-Term-Care www.techforltc.org

e) Vandoren Saxophone Harness

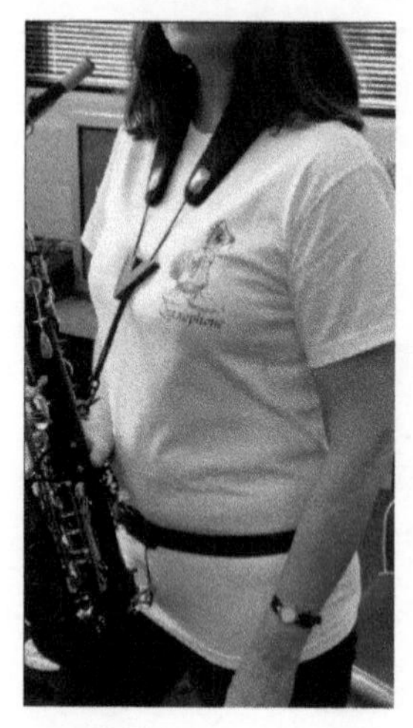

Source: www.sax.co.uk

Features:

Shoulder straps soft and handmade, these take pressure off your neck and distribute it. The instrument cord secures your instrument discreetly, without uncomfortable straps that restrict your breathing. Stabilizing rods work independently as you move and these give you leverage to offset your instrument's weight. The support belt centers the load at your waist, balancing you perfectly whether standing or sitting. Universal fit suitable for any saxophone, and can be sized to fit children and adults.

Indications:

- Rotator cuff injuries

Where to Buy: www.sax.co.uk

f) Long Handle Shoe Horn

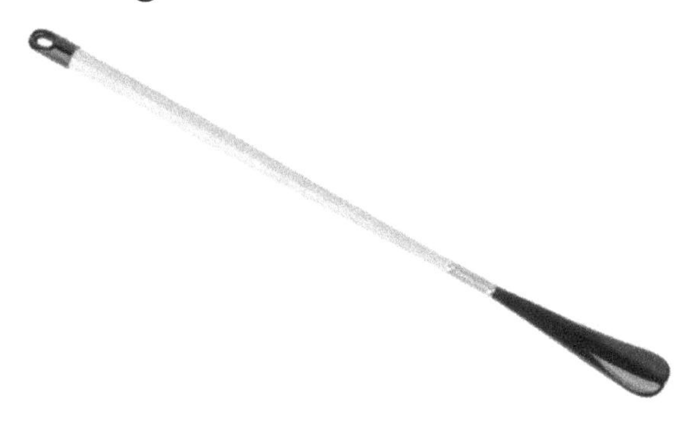

Source: www.amazon.com

Features:

Long Handle Shoe Horn facilitates putting shoes on easier, with less effort.

It is available in various sizes ranging from 24 to 31 inches.

No bending or twisting is required. Hence it is most suitable for people with back and shoulder injuries.

Indications:

- Rotator cuff injuries

- Back pain

Where to Buy:

Pair Arm-Extender X-Long Shoe Horns Big Handle 19" –

www.ebay.com

Long Handle 23"Easy to use stainless steel shoehorn –

31" Long Handle Shoe Horn www.amazon.com

Index

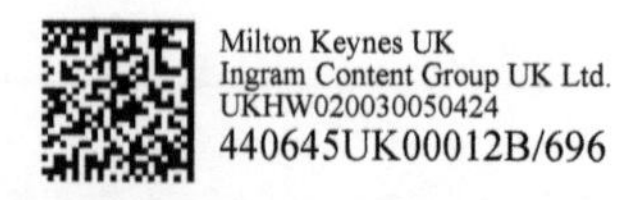
Milton Keynes UK
Ingram Content Group UK Ltd.
UKHW020030050424
440645UK00012B/696

9 781909 151710